THE COMMON SENSE GUIDE TO

IMPROVING PALLIATIVE CARE

Joanne Lynn

Ekta Chaudhry

Lin Noyes Simon

Anne M. Wilkinson

Janice Lynch Schuster

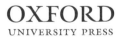
OXFORD
UNIVERSITY PRESS

2007

OXFORD
UNIVERSITY PRESS

Oxford University Press, Inc., publishes works that further
Oxford University's objective of excellence
in research, scholarship, and education.

Oxford   New York
Auckland   Cape Town   Dar es Salaam   Hong Kong   Karachi
Kuala Lumpur   Madrid   Melbourne   Mexico City   Nairobi
New Delhi   Shanghai   Taipei   Toronto

With offices in
Argentina   Austria   Brazil   Chile   Czech Republic   France   Greece
Guatemala   Hungary   Italy   Japan   Poland   Portugal   Singapore
South Korea   Switzerland   Thailand   Turkey   Ukraine   Vietnam

Copyright © 2007 by Oxford University Press

Published by Oxford University Press, Inc.
198 Madison Avenue, New York, New York 10016

www.oup.com

Oxford is a registered trademark of Oxford University Press

Library of Congress Cataloging-in-Publication Data
The common sense guide to improving palliative care / Joanne Lynn . . . [et al.].
      p. ; cm.
   Includes bibliographical references and index.
   ISBN-13 978-0-19-531041-2
   ISBN 0-19-531041-1
   1. Palliative treatment.   2. Hospice care.   I. Lynn, Joanne, 1951–
   [DNLM: 1. Palliative Care—organization & administration—United States.
2. Quality Assurance, Health Care—methods—United States.   3. Terminal Care—
organization & administration—United States. WB 310 C734 2007]
   R726.8.C66 2007
   616'.029—dc22   2006012754

9 8 7 6 5 4 3 2 1

Printed in the United States of America
on acid-free paper

THE COMMON SENSE GUIDE TO

IMPROVING PALLIATIVE CARE

Preface

This guide is for clinicians and managers hoping to improve the care that people living in the shadow of death can count on. This guide distills what we have learned from working with a few hundred clinical teams across the United States and abroad. With the pointers given here, nurses, physicians, or administrators can set about making their local care system into a reliably high-quality service to support seriously ill people and their families.

This short guide has a companion volume, *Improving Care for the End of Life* (Oxford University Press, rev. ed., 2007), which includes many more tools, improvement strategies, references, and narratives from specific teams making improvements in care for the last stages of life. We also recommend updated information from the U.S. Medicare quality-improvement projects (http://www.medqic.org), from worldwide private efforts to improve health care quality (http://www.ihi.org), from the Center to Advance Palliative Care (http://www.capc.org), and from our own work on quality improvement (http://www.medicaring.org).

This book has had many supporters, and we are grateful to the clinical teams who have so generously taught us so much. We thank the RAND Corporation for providing a home to the Palliative Care Policy Center, both for our research endeavors and our quality improvement initiatives. We also want to thank the Kaiser Foundation Research Institute, the Dr. Sidney Garfield Memorial Fund, and Catholic Health Care West, California, for providing financial support to enable us to write the guide and to the Retirement Research Foundation and the Alfred P. Sloan Foundation for the support that first enabled us to write *Improving Care for the End of Life*. All who use rapid-cycle methods are indebted to the Institute for Healthcare Improvement for its vision of better care at the end of life. We thank Oxford University Press for the guidance that it has provided for this book and for its substantial commitment to publishing in palliative care. We thank the Quality and Access Division at the National Hospice and Palliative Care Organization and Diane Meier of the Center to Advance Palliative Care for their review of drafts of sections of this book. Finally, we thank Lisa Spear for attending to the details of preparing the manuscript and Les Morgan for revising it to appear on the Inter-Institutional Collaborating Network for Palliative Care, which is available online at many sites (including http://www.medicaring.org and http://www.growthhouse.org).

Chapter 12 is based largely on the writings of Diane Meier, MD, FACP, Director of the Center to Advance Palliative Care at Mount Sinai School of Medicine, and Charles von Gunten, MD, PhD, FACP, Director of the Center for Palliative Studies, San Diego Hospice and Palliative Care (see also http://www.capc.org).

CONTENTS

1 An Orientation 3

2 Basics of Quality Improvement 21

3 Advance Care Planning 43

4 Preventing, Assessing, and Treating Pain 61

5 Assuring Comfort 77

6 Caring for Caregivers 95

7 Continuity and Transfers 117

8 Chronic Care: Heart and Lung Failure 137

9 Nursing Home Quality: Pressure Ulcers 153

10 Improving Care for People with Advanced Dementia 173
and Their Families

11 Improving Intensive Care Units 191

12 Building a Palliative Care Program 205

13 Hospice Program Quality 221

14 End-of-Life Care, Spiritual Support, and Bereavement 233

15 Beyond Quality Improvement: Policy Improvement 249

Index 259

THE COMMON SENSE GUIDE TO

IMPROVING PALLIATIVE CARE

An Orientation

Healthcare is changing for the better for patients nearing the end of life. Changes being tested and tried by organizations nationwide demonstrate that we can and must make life better for people with advanced, and eventually fatal, illnesses. Using a rapid-cycle approach to quality improvement (QI), hundreds of teams have found that straightforward approaches to complex problems can actually lead to improvements for patients and families. In the midst of the physical and emotional suffering that often accompany dying, these teams have found that they can comfort the sick; that pain and a score of other symptoms can be managed; that advance care plans can be located and honored; that transfers can be almost seamless; and, certainly, that human relationships can be strengthened. Although it may take some time to design and implement a program of one's own, the process is easy to understand and follow; it is simple enough to try one or two changes with one or two patients and then go on from there, as other groups have. For instance, consider the following examples.

- A California skilled-nursing facility found that only 26% of their residents had a documented advance directive. An improvement team decided to do better. They gave patients and families very clear instructions about life-sustaining treatments and what it meant to use each of them. The team created a process to transfer records from the facility to other hospitals and clinics in its system, ensuring that advance directives went along. And they added completion of the advance directive to the weekly interdisciplinary team meeting, including it as a goal for every patient. Within six months, 70% of their patients had a documented advance directive at discharge; within 10 months, 91% did. Three months later, the level remained this high, and everyone at the facility had come to expect that a documented advance directive was simply part of good care.

- A volunteer meal-delivery program wanted to expand the scope of its work to offer prevention services along with hot meals. Its QI team aimed to reduce falls among its elderly clients by assessing homes for safety issues and ensuring that someone had made the necessary changes within six months. In the target group, only one client was hospitalized for a fall, compared to 36% of clients in a similar group who did not get the services. After that success, the group decided to add a two-hour visit with patients by a social worker to screen for depression. The social worker found that 60% of the clients reported feeling depressed; and, of these, 75% said they had no one to turn to in an emergency. The project recruited volunteers to make twice-weekly phone calls to their clients, using a discussion of menu choices for Meals on Wheels as the reason for the call. These calls provided regular social contact for the clients and current information about client needs to the program. The endeavor delighted both the homebound clients and the volunteers.

- A major urban hospital realized that many patients returned to their hospital beds without having completed scheduled diagnostic tests because they were in too much pain. At first, nurses were told to "try harder" to assess pain, but this brought about no real improvement. Then, the radiology department decided to give transport orderlies training in using a pain intensity scale. Orderlies were instructed not to transport a patient unless the nurse on duty had completed the form and, if necessary, had treated the patient's pain. This process resulted in huge changes: the number of patients assessed and treated for pain before undergoing a diagnostic test went from 16 to 92%. Within a few months, *no* patients were returned to the unit because they were in too much pain to undergo a test. Today, this process is standard procedure throughout the hospital. The hospital views it as an adverse event if a patient is returned because pain prevented a diagnostic test.

- Because of travel time, a hospice found that each nurse was able to admit only one or two patients per day. The hospice decided to train other staff to perform most of the admissions work, especially the duties of contacting and visiting families to explain the hospice benefit. This freed nurses to see three or four patients daily and increased by 37% the number of patients admitted to hospice within 24 hours of referral.

These groups sound so good, you might think that we made them up. But in fact, people like you, eager to improve how palliative care is done, created these stories with hard work and dedication. Like them, you too can use rapid-cycle QI methods to make substantial changes. You can use these methods in any healthcare setting, and you can do so quickly, effectively, and efficiently. This manual shows you how to jump start QI, no matter where you work, so as to improve your organization's practices. We focus on patients with advanced illness and those coming to the end of life, though the QI method works in other populations as well.

Everyone wants to improve healthcare, and many even have great ideas for doing so. Sometimes, the toughest part can be figuring out where to start and forging the will to get changes underway. We will show you how to develop a QI project, measure what you are doing, figure out whether what you have tried really leads to improvement, and sustain the improvements that you achieve.

BETTER CARE FOR PATIENTS AND FAMILIES: MAKE IT HAPPEN

Many clinical teams with whom we have partnered have focused on one or more of four areas that are well tested and offer good starting points. Eventually, you may want to work on all four areas. At first, though, focus on the one area that seems to cause the greatest distress for patients in your care—and on one that seems changeable for the better. Most groups find that they can do the following.

- Improve comfort by preventing or treating pain, shortness of breath, pressure ulcers, and other symptoms.
- Enhance continuity of care by reducing unnecessary transfers and being sure to transfer the care plan with advance directives. Generally, people should be able to die "in place," where they live.
- Improve advance care planning so that everyone involved in caring for a patient is aware of preferences and decisions about treatments, including ventilation, nutrition, hydration, and plans for care.
- Attend to the emotional and spiritual needs of patients and families, from the practical (Are you still sending bills to the deceased patient?) to the spiritual (Does the patient want to see a clergy member or spiritual adviser) to the emotional

(Do you know what a patient needs to feel happy as life draws to an end?).

Here, you will find practical information about how to make such improvements. At the most general level, effective improvement requires the following:

- a QI *team*;
- a clear and significant *aim*;
- a way to *measure,* track, and report progress;
- a list of *changes* worth trying;
- the *will to improve* within your organization.

QI: WHY YOU NEED TO GIVE IT A TRY

In its 2001 report, *Crossing the Quality Chasm: A New Health System for the 21st Century,* the Institute of Medicine sets six aims that all healthcare providers can use to improve the healthcare environment:

1. *Safe,* one that avoid injuries;
2. *Effective,* with services based on scientific knowledge and offered only to those likely to benefit from them;
3. *Patient-centered,* offering care that is respectful of and responsive to the patient;
4. *Timely,* reducing waits and harmful delays;
5. *Efficient,* avoiding waste of equipment, supplies, ideas, and energy;
6. *Equitable,* offering care that does not vary in character because of patient characteristics (such as gender, age, or race).

Quality improvement has the obvious benefit of improved patient care in all settings, and it has long been mandated for hospital and nursing home licensure. Now hospices and even physicians' offices are implementing QI practices.

How to Start Changing Practices

When Elisabeth Kübler-Ross set out to study dying people in the late 1960s in her own university hospital, clinicians responded that they had no patient known to be dying! Ignoring reality is often easier than acknowledging it or changing it. Today, many healthcare organizations tend to believe that they actually have little need to change: everyone else might need to change and improve, but *we* are doing just fine. However, many more groups now admit that they may not be doing a perfect job and want to do better.

The first thing you will need to do is to understand what is not working in your system and why. You will need a clear picture of the current situation and how you can improve practices. Take a close look at what your organization is already doing in any of the usual target areas: pain and symptom management, advance care planning, transfers and continuity, and psychosocial/spiritual support for patients and families. Consider your current practices by asking a few pointed questions such as these:

- Do we know each patient's pain score?
- How many patients are in pain 48, 24, or 4 hours before death?
- Do families report that patients die in pain?
- Can we locate advance directives in less than one hour?
- Did issues come up over ventilator use or its discontinuation?
- Do families have conflicts or regrets about the care that their loved one received prior to death?
- How many frail, elderly patients endured CPR before death?
- How many were recent transfers from nursing homes?
- Did patients (and families) have a chance to meet with a spiritual adviser?
- Did families receive support while keeping vigil for a relative?

- Are families participating in bereavement programs? How many families do so? Do we know how families are doing six months after the patient's death?

These questions seem pretty straightforward. But when groups are asked to take a hard look at what is usual and routine in their settings, they tend to be shocked by what they find. Consider the following examples.

- One hospice found that one-half of the the patients being admitted had pain intensity levels greater than five (on a 0–10 scale).
- One hospital learned that a complaint of severe pain led to an average of one hour to get an assessment and orders and then another two hours before administration of a changed medication, so hospital patients in pain were averaging a three-hour wait!
- Another hospital found that one-half of its attending physicians did not register to prescribe controlled substances and thus could not write prescriptions at discharge for patients with serious pain in order to cover the time until the patients were resettled at home.

On the one hand, uncovering these shortcomings can make you want to throw in the towel. On the other, leaders intent on QI see these problems as opportunities to strive for excellence. Improvement starts with "What is wrong?" and "What if?" questions and then moves ahead when clinicians decide to take action on behalf of their patients.

The rapid-cycle QI method can quickly improve patient care. Such change does not require congressional action or discussion by the hospital's board of directors: improvement simply requires dedicated people working toward an aim that is important to patients and families.

Our work has most often engaged QI groups from hospitals (most often emergency rooms, intensive care units, and acute care), nursing homes, home health agencies, and hospices. Their patients, clients, and residents range from those in the early stages of a serious illness to those in their final days before death. Each of these situations requires different types of change, so we have varied our examples. Each chapter includes suggestions about adapting interventions to particular environments and to the specific needs of patients and families living with serious illness or of those passing through the hours and days just before death.

Once you have made improvements, you will want your colleagues to adopt these QI methods and to expand the scope of your intervention. This will lead to the next step in the improvement process: testing interventions on ever-larger groups or in different settings. Some teams have been so successful that their strategies have spread throughout their entire system or community. Of course, this is hard work. If it were easy, it would already be done. Sometimes, you may find that you have to go back a few times even to establish an aim that anchors the work.

QI teams like yours, nationwide, have discovered that their work in improving care for advanced chronic illness patients and those at the end of life has benefits for other patients and providers in their own healthcare system. Moreover, some improve delivery of healthcare throughout their region and among different care providers. As discussed at the beginning of this chapter, teams have achieved important goals within just a few months.

This manual features practical, hands-on skills and techniques to help you do just that. Each chapter features steps on how to get started; how to develop, test, and measure changes; and how to spread your ideas. Each chapter includes stories based on the experiences and achievements of the groups with which we have worked. These stories show you how others have accomplished improvement and inspire the confidence that you can change things for the better. This manual will also provide ready-to-use ideas for change, as well as tools with which to measure improvement.

THE POWER OF PROMISES

In the care of very sick people, the error is not that we *never* provide good care; it is that we do not *always* provide good care. One particularly strong way to envision a really good care system is to imagine a clinician sitting down with a patient and family who face a serious, and eventually fatal, condition. What would the patient and family want the clinician to be able to promise, right through to the end of life? You can cover most of what people in the last phase of life want from their healthcare in these seven promises (Lynn, 2004, p.22):

1. evidence-based, appropriate medical treatment;
2. no overwhelming symptoms;
3. continuity of comprehensive care;
4. planning ahead for complications and death;
5. care customized to the patient's preferences;
6. care adapted to serve the patient's family;
7. help to live as fully as possible.

In deciding on their improvement priorities, many teams find it useful to ask, "What keeps us from making these promises?" The idea of keeping promises is highly motivating, and it targets all goals toward high reliability.

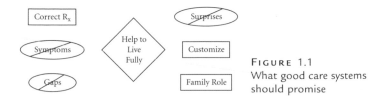

FIGURE 1.1
What good care systems
should promise

Others have done it, and you can, too. As you improve the ways in which your organization cares for patients and families, we ask you to take action to change the larger system of care, not only in your community but nationally, too. As you know, the care system too often fails patients and families. This guide will enable you to become a force for change in how we care for people with advanced chronic illness and near the end of life.

The Temporarily Immortal and the Dying: Who's Who?

The boundary between those who are healthy (or merely chronically ill) and those who are dying is not obvious, yet we often link appropriate care to that transition between categories. It is well worth taking some time to consider what truth there is in that distinction. We talk about the living and the dying as if the difference were obvious, as obvious as the distinction between men and women. But deciding who is dying is more subjective than that; it is more like the distinctions between short and tall or thin and heavy. As long as we—patients, families, caregivers, clinicians—are pursuing a cure or even a return to better health, we count ourselves as being among the living, the "temporarily immortal." Once we accept that the situation will worsen and that treatment will be futile, then we join the dying. Most of us would prefer to be counted among the dying only for a short time at the end of life, not for years and years, as happens when we need palliative care for a long time.

However, life and death are not that simple. Many people with serious and eventually fatal illness continue to function in their usual social roles. Eventually, the combination of multiple illnesses and the frailty of advanced age lead to increasing disability and, after perhaps five years, eventual death. The usual course toward the end of life is a number of years of increasing disease, disability, and use of healthcare services; the situation, then, is no longer an either/or proposition. Most do not look as though they are dying, and they would not describe themselves that way, either. The rather misleading way we think about "the dying" frames much of our public policy and healthcare. The Medicare hospice benefit, for instance, requires that patients have a "life expectancy of six months or less if the disease takes its normal course" (42 CFR Part 418, p. 916). Many laws about living wills, forgoing life-sustaining treatment, and advance directives use the term "terminal illness." Often, these policies serve to exclude people with desperate needs but ambiguous prognoses, especially people who are stable but in very fragile condition.

When trying to label patients as appropriate for hospice or palliative care (or not), organizations need to begin by redefining their terms. Rather than focusing on those who are clearly "dying," we need to consider patients for whom increasing illness and disability will lead to death sometime in the next few years and to think about how to offer them the kinds of services that help patients live well, even while dying. We have come to use the "surprise" question, first tested by Franciscan Health Services in Washington State: ask clinicians, "Would you be surprised if this patient died in the next six months or so?" Those whose death would not be surprising need palliative care, or at least advance care planning, comfort care, and psychosocial support. However, defining the population in this way means that there is no clear time when the patient gets *only* treatment or *only* palliation. Some patients will need both ICU care and do-not-resuscitate (DNR) decisions; some will want to be on transplant lists *and* record an oral history for a family legacy. Some who are sick enough to die will die within days, but others may hang on for years.

WHAT IS PALLIATIVE CARE? WHY IS IT NOT HOSPICE?

Throughout this manual, we will talk about *palliative care*, a term with many official definitions and sometimes confusing meanings. We generally use the definition from the World Health Organization, which calls it "the active total care of patients whose disease is not responsive to curative treatment . . . [when] control of pain, of other symptoms, and of psychological, social, and spiritual problems is paramount" (WHO, 1990). People who receive palliative care may receive disease-modifying and comfort measures simultaneously, and they may require such care for years.

Hospice, however, is the term used to describe an array of services provided to patients close to dying. In the United States, hospice tends to be defined by the Medicare hospice benefit, which requires that the patient's prognosis is to live six months or less. This prognostic requirement often prevents hospice providers from caring for stable patients with advanced illnesses such as heart and lung failure, dementia, or frailty, which can have persistently uncertain prognoses. Palliative care usually serves a broader period of time.

Trajectories of Illness: Matching the Care System to How People Die

For the most part, we tend to organize different approaches to care of the dying around providers of services: hospitals, nursing homes, hospices, and private homes. Or, we organize care by specific diseases. But the reality is that either kind of organizational scheme ensures that people often do not get the care they need, when they most need it, and in an environment that makes sense. The conventional divisions, by disease and setting of care, do not work well because most patients with fatal conditions have multiple diseases and disabilities that require multiple care settings.

In the last few years, healthcare providers and organizations, as well as policymakers and public officials, have started to think about organizing services based on the trajectories that people follow when living with a fatal illness. Within the population of people with serious, progressive, and eventually fatal chronic illnesses are three subcategories: patients with a short period of evident decline, often from cancer; patients with long-term limitations with intermittent serious episodes, mostly heart and lung failure; and patients with prolonged dwindling, such as frailty and dementia. Each of these three pathways to dying presents its own challenges and requirements. Cancer patients, for instance, benefit from intense but relatively brief hospice care, while patients who have organ system failure require long-term standby support to live with their uncertain prognosis. Those who succumb to frailty and dementia will need intensely personal care through a long period of dependency. Figure 1.2 shows the three trajectories.

People at this final stage of life still want to live as well as possible and for as long as possible. They and their families have many goals: relief from symptoms, help with family burdens, control of personal expenditures for healthcare, keeping a high quality of life, being in control and maintaining dignity, and having an opportunity to come to peace with spiritual issues and relationships. These goals coexist with those of preventing illness and prolonging life, even when pursuing such goals requires aggressive or invasive treatments. Pursuing these goals simultaneously contrasts with the usual thinking that people near death need comfort and closure but not treatment. Instead of a transition from cure to care, people living with fatal chronic illnesses have many complex goals and priorities that evolve over time.

For people engaged in QI, this conceptual model is a way to see the forest *and* the trees. Becoming aware of the trajectories allows us to tailor services to match. People with congestive heart failure, for instance, often assume that they will always be rescued from exacerbations and live. If they realize instead that death will likely be rather sudden, they might see the importance of naming a healthcare proxy and expressing their preferences for end-of-life care. Families are often surprised when a loved one dies from lung failure, because no one has

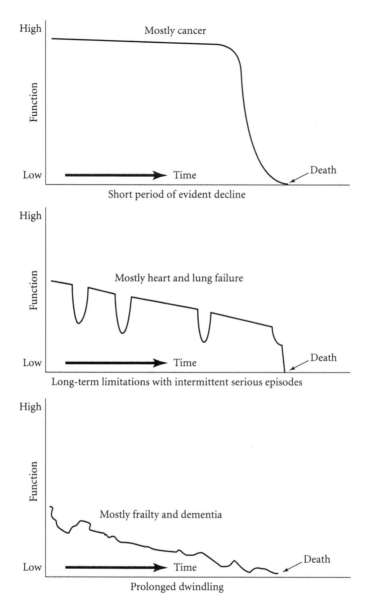

FIGURE 1.2 Chronic illness in the elderly typically follows one of three trajectories. Copyright 2003, RAND Corp. Reprinted with permission.

told them that this is the likely end. Healthcare professionals must reassess these practices and develop more appropriate patterns of care.

As people progress through their illness trajectory, they will have changing needs for assistance which, in turn, produce changing demands on family caregivers. Below are three lists detailing a number of issues important to caregivers of patients within each of the three trajectories.

Advanced Cancer

- Comfort and symptom management affecting the patient's quality of life (e.g., pain, depression, fatigue, breathlessness, and so forth).
- Accurate and timely information, support, and assistance before and after a loved one's death.
- Fairly rapid decline and death pose poignant but often difficult opportunities for farewells.

Advanced Organ System Failure

- An erratic disease course requiring complex management and changing levels of caregiving, with sometimes intense, hands-on care interspersed with periods of relative calm.
- The continual potential for unexpected death in the context of the often unacknowledged fatal disease.
- Physicians, family, and patient often do not acknowledge the fatal nature of the illness.

Advanced Dementia

- Altered behavior and personality in patient can be stressful for loved ones, who need help learning how to cope and respond.
- Family must make decisions, often difficult, on behalf of the patients.

- Families may need to decide to place a loved one in a nursing home, usually a wrenching decision.
- Can require long-term caregiving, often for years and often challenging.

Looking for Improvement Everywhere

Improvement in care for advanced illness and the end of life will ultimately require multiple perspectives, many approaches to change, and the joint efforts of biomedical researchers, policymakers, healthcare professionals, and the public. However, reform will almost certainly begin with you: a healthcare professional, paraprofessional, administrator, or chief executive oficer, someone who realizes that what is going on should not go on, and someone who is willing to take a chance on change.

Most of us alive today—you, and those you love—are lucky. Unlike previous generations, the majority of us will grow old and die late in life of chronic illness. As we age, we will turn to the healthcare system for information, care, and support. In its current setup, that system will fail. Those with advanced chronic illness or near the end of life suffer from pain and other physical symptoms, from fear and confusion, from isolation and uncertainty. We know that this is so, and we know that we can change it. We should start now, with four or five patients in our care, by picking something we can make better. We promise that you can and will and that your efforts will lead to better care—and better lives and deaths for your patients. We have an unprecedented opportunity to improve the system, to make a difference in how people die, not only in the next decade, but in the next year. Such opportunities to make a difference are rare, and if we do not make the most of them now, we will find ourselves dying in the wasteful and unreliable system we allowed to drift along.

Give Them Something to Talk About

Better care for advanced chronic illness and the end of life demands profound changes in how we design, finance, and deliver healthcare for people with advanced chronic and life-threatening illnesses; first, it demands leaders who can envision better care and take steps to achieve it. Dividing the "dying" from the living and providing palliative care only to those who clearly are dying is an approach that prevents us from developing comprehensive systems of care for all seriously ill patients as they move from health to disability and eventual death.

Rapid-cycle changes for QI can create real and lasting improvement in most organizations in less than one year. Many healthcare organizations have used this approach to make significant strides in how they care for patients with advanced chronic illness and near the end of life. You will, too, so let us get started.

References

42 CFR Part 418, Text from Code of Federal Regulations. Available from U.S. Government Printing Office at http://www.gpoaccess.gov/cfr/index.html

Committee on Quality of Health Care in America, Institute of Medicine. (2001). *Crossing the Quality Chasm: A New Health System for the 21st Century.* Washington, DC: National Academy Press.

Kübler-Ross, E. (1969/1997). *On Death and Dying.* New York: Simon and Schuster.

Lynn, J. (2004). *Sick to Death and Not Going to Take It Anymore! Reforming Health Care for the Last Years of Life.* Berkeley: University of California Press.

World Health Organization (WHO). (1990). Cancer Pain Relief and Palliative Care. Report of WHO Expert Committee, Technical Series No. 804. Geneva: WHO.

2

Basics of Quality Improvement

In This Chapter

- Starting a quality-improvement project
- Finding the right people for your project
- Sustaining your success
- Spreading your success throughout the organization

Wanting to improve the quality of care in your organization is a great idea: but how do you do it? This manual, based on the examples of scores of other groups, offers ideas and tips so that you can literally get started tomorrow. Before tackling specific issues, such as advance care planning or pain management, take time to review the basics of rapid-cycle quality improvement (QI), a well-tested and efficient method for making deliberate improvements in care. This model was developed for use in healthcare by the Boston-based Institute for Healthcare Improvement (IHI), which provides many resources, including breakthrough series programs, conference calls, and an extensive website.

Rapid-cycle QI requires teams to set aims, try out changes, and measure the effects in order to decide what to do next. To get started, you need to answer three questions:

1. What are we trying to accomplish? (Aim)
2. What can we do to improve things? (Changes)

3. How will we know that the change is an improvement?
   (Measures)

With answers to these questions in mind, your team will stay focused and move forward quickly. Try writing down your answers to these questions right now, and then use the rest of this chapter to sharpen your answers and shape your project. Once you have answered these questions, the QI method tests your ideas and tracks your progress. The rest of this chapter explains how to make the process work.

Identifying the Problem and Stating Your Aim

Most teams want to jump right in to identify issues and nominate fixes for the most prominent problems affecting their patients or clients. But this jump-start can lock you into misplaced priorities. It is usually better to have your group do some brainstorming and a little research to identify real problems (i.e., patterns of service delivery that create problems for patients and families) and to consider which to tackle first. You may have to collect some data—just a bit—to check your hunches. For instance, you might not think pain management is an issue for your organization, until you discover that it takes several hours to get medication from the pharmacy to the floor.

Once you think that you know what the problem is, check to be sure. At the same time, do not let indecision slow you down; rather, be committed to getting started . . . now! Our favorite mantra is, "What can you do by next Tuesday?"—a question that pushes you to get started with what is at hand. By next Tuesday, you can probably try out a pain scale for dementia patients, test an advance care planning checklist for nursing home residents and families, or put together a hospitality cart for families keeping vigil in the intensive care unit.

With the problem reasonably well identified, you will next develop an aim.

WHAT ARE WE TRYING TO ACCOMPLISH? (WRITING AN EFFECTIVE AIM)

This sounds like an easy task, doesn't it? Actually, writing an aim can become challenging, but a few pointers will get you there. First, write down what you want to accomplish. Keep it simple, as in the following examples:

> *General Statement: Improve advance care planning for the patients in this particular hospital unit.*

Or:

> *Provide better pain management for all of our cancer patients.*

Once you have a general statement, you will need to convert it into a useful aim.

Elements of Effective Aims

1. What will improve?
2. When will it improve?
3. How much will it improve?
4. For whom will it improve?

Take a look at an aim statement that includes all of the four components.

> *Aim Statement: In 30 days, 90% of inpatient cancer patients on unit 4A will report pain levels lower than their own pain goal by the evening shift on their second hospital day.*

This example features the four components needed to set a focused and clear aim. Anyone who reads this statement will be able to understand what you are trying to accomplish in your project, and the aim statement will keep your team focused and on track.

> **What will improve:** *Pain management should be brought within the patient's acceptable range within one day.*
> **When:** *Within 30 days of project start.*
> **How much:** *Increase from 30% at baseline to 90%.*
> **For whom:** *Inpatient cancer patients on unit 4A.*

Coming up with a useful aim is hard to do. You have to clarify your goals, think how you will measure them, and make it enough of stretch to be worth doing. Try not to use the QI model for tiny gains; teams actually stay enthused for the work more readily if the goal is obviously worthwhile and clearly an improvement. Be prepared to adjust your aim as you work through the other issues, such as establishing a team and developing a process, which we describe in this chapter.

ESTABLISHING A GOOD TEAM

Having the right people on the team—which may mean including people from other areas of your organization—is key to your success. Shortcomings in healthcare processes almost always involve multiple people. Few important changes can be implemented by a single individual; you need a group to make it happen. You probably have colleagues who also see problems and are willing to work to correct them. These are the first few people you should consider to enlist for your team.

Get together with them and forge the commitment to make changes. Describe your ideas about possible aims, and ask for their thoughts on other goals.

Once you have the general goal settled, think about the kinds of expertise the team will need. If you are working on pain, you may need a pharmacist. If you are working on the transfer of advance care plans, you may need admissions clerks. Try to include people whose expertise covers the four areas described below, and you will be on your way to having an effective team. (Remember, however, that one person may play several roles.)

ORGANIZATION LEADER Invite someone who has enough clout to insist on the changes you want to test and who can help you get the time and resources you will need. For example, bring in the vice president for patient services or the director of palliative medicine. This person may not attend all team meetings, but it really helps to have a leader who understands the importance of the project, can help with personnel or resource issues, and is up-to-date on its progress.

CONTENT EXPERT Someone on the team has to have the clinical knowledge about your problem area and a thorough understanding of care processes in your system. This person is most likely a clinician who is also a champion for the improvement team. This "clinical champion" can guide the team and also engage other clinicians.

IMPROVEMENT EXPERT You need someone with expertise in improvement methods to help the team implement the QI model. Many of the tools and processes of teamwork, measurement, and implementation are applicable across all sorts of improvement activities. This person can be someone from the QI department, if your organization has one. With the help of this book, you, too, will become an improvement expert.

TEAM LEADER This person drives the project on a day-to-day basis. The team leader understands the details of the system and makes sure work is getting done. A nurse manager, pharmacist, or clinical social worker often takes on this role, but background does not matter as much as whether the person is willing to commit to the project and stay with it.

Very often, this is the person who makes sure that meetings happen, updates are sent out, and data are collected.

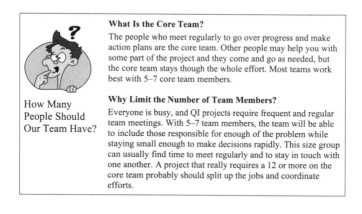

How Many
People Should
Our Team Have?

What Is the Core Team?
The people who meet regularly to go over progress and make action plans are the core team. Other people may help you with some part of the project and they come and go as needed, but the core team stays though the whole effort. Most teams work best with 5–7 core team members.

Why Limit the Number of Team Members?
Everyone is busy, and QI projects require frequent and regular team meetings. With 5–7 team members, the team will be able to include those responsible for enough of the problem while staying small enough to make decisions rapidly. This size group can usually find time to meet regularly and to stay in touch with one another. A project that really requires a 12 or more on the core team probably should split up the jobs and coordinate efforts.

The team leader needs to keep the team motivated and draw on the strength of each team member. To prevent and resolve any conflict that may arise among your team, try the following.

1. Ensure that members agree on the aim.
2. Identify areas of agreement within the team regarding its work.
3. Determine if the differences within the team are actually interfering with its work. If so, then try to resolve those differences.
4. Decide which issue is most problematic for the team as a whole and discuss alternative ways of accomplishing your goals.
5. Keep up enthusiasm by getting positive statements from patients and managers back to the team or by pointing out successes.

Everyone on the team should have a clear understanding of who is doing what and then arrive at meetings with their assigned task done.

It is good to ask for a commitment from each team member in which they agree to be involved for the duration of the project. Even in environments where there is high staff turnover, role delineation is important. If a team member does leave, the project need not lose steam: Find another person to join, and assume the duties and tasks of the person who has left. For QI teams, the tasks to cover include the following:

- Who will implement the changes?
- Who will tell other people about changes to be tried?
- Who will collect and analyze the data? Who will plot and track changes for a storyboard?
- Who will keep senior leaders in the loop and informed of your progress or need for additional resources?
- Who will run the meetings, write the agenda and the minutes (if necessary), and keep a to-do list?

Although people tend to shy away from conflict, encourage team members to talk about their concerns. You want everybody to participate, not just those who speak first or loudest. Of course, conflict is unacceptable if it is about personalities. Agree on some ground rules for team behavior, including the following:

- Attend meetings, be prepared, and arrive on time.
- Have an agenda and stick to it.
- End meetings on time.
- No cell phones, chatting, or side conversations are allowed during the team meetings.
- Speak respectfully and bring up problems during the meeting, and speak up about your concerns.
- Do not denigrate the team or its work in front of colleagues.
- If you know you are going to be too busy to accomplish your assigned task, discuss it in the meeting and get help so that the whole project is not delayed.

MEASURING YOUR SUCCESS

Now you need to work on the critical question: How will we know that our change is an improvement? In our example, How will we know when cancer patients have their pain level lower than their pain goal by the end of their second hospital day? The simplest answer is by measuring your progress.

How do we decide what to measure? The answer lies in our aim statement: implicit in the aim is the way to measure your success.

Let us use the previous example to identify a measurement strategy. Remember the aim:

> **Aim Statement:** *In 30 days, 90% of inpatient cancer patients on unit 4A will report pain levels lower than their own pain goal by the evening shift of their second hospital day.*

One measure to chart the progress of this aim statement is the percentage of all cancer patients on unit 4A who have pain levels lower than their stated pain goal by the evening shift of the second hospital day. In this example, the numerator is the number of patients with pain who meet their pain goal, and the denominator is all cancer patients with pain on admission. Try to link your measurement strategy to your aim. Make it practical and important. Each chapter in this book provides suggestions about measurement strategies that work. There are three types of measures: outcomes, process, and adverse effects.

OUTCOME MEASURES   An outcome measure seeks an accurate means of assessing directly what you care about most, such as the patient/family experience.

Using our pain example, an outcome measure is the percentage of all cancer patients with pain on unit 4A who have pain levels lower than their stated pain goals by the evening shift of the second hospital day. (Levels are based on a scale of 0–10.)

To calculate this measure, you need to know how many cancer patients had pain on admission and stayed until the evening of their second hospital day; of these, you must record how many had pain below their own target by the evening shift of their second hospital day. A cancer patient who has no pain on admission would not be included in the denominator. Notice that this way of specifying the measure would miss postoperative pain on the third hospital day and also patients who died or went home in a day. Like most measurement strategies, you have to pick a specific measure that best relates to your aim. Working on your measure often requires that you go back and sharpen your aim.

PROCESS MEASURES A process measure assesses how your care delivery system is working. Do certain desirable actions happen in the right order and at the right time?

Using our pain example, some process measures would be as follows.

- Percentage of cancer patients on unit 4A with documentation of pain assessment and their acceptable pain level within four hours of admission (level of pain, pain goal).
- Percentage of cancer patients with pain on unit 4A with documentation of treatment for their pain within 24 hours of admission.
- Percentage of cancer patients on unit 4A with documentation of pain greater than five (on a 0–10 scale) who have revised treatment administered within one hour.

Improved pain management in cancer patients requires looking at the steps in the process to identify, treat, and reassess pain in the patients on unit 4A. Are patients being assessed for pain when they are admitted to the unit, and, once assessed, are they being treated? Once treated, are they being reassessed? These process measures are important and often are easier to determine than outcome measures, partly because they happen more often. The major concern with relying only on process measures is whether they are tightly linked to the outcome you really care about. Often, team members will measure processes just long enough to be sure that they are working correctly, but they will keep measuring outcomes until they achieve the aim.

ADVERSE EFFECTS Changes that you make in the patterns of care often result in adverse effects. For example, having nurses spend time doing pain assessment, treatment, and reassessment on unit 4A may result in longer waiting times for patients in the emergency room to move to unit 4A. You need to monitor likely or important side effects while keeping surveillance on the project's overall effects.

To choose a measurement strategy, we suggest the following.

1. Look at what other teams have used (see chapters in this manual, or consult other professional publications on QI).
2. Measure outcomes whenever you can.
3. Simplify measurement whenever possible; for example, sample one shift, ask just one or two questions, or piggyback on another measurement instrument that is already in use.
4. Start out measuring a few things, and let some drop if they are too difficult or not informative enough, and use other, more responsive measures.
4. Measure a process just long enough to be sure that the improvement is in place.

Here is another example.

> **Aim statement:** *Within six months, 85% of congestive heart failure (CHF) or chronic obstructive pulmonary disease (COPD) patients in our outpatient clinic will have advance care plans (addressing such key issues as CPR, surrogate intervention, and ventilator use) completed and documented in their electronic medical record.*

What will improve: Advance care planning.

When: Within six months.

By how much: Eighty-five percent of patients, up from current estimates of "occasional."

For whom: Clinic CHF/COPD patients.

Outcome Measure: The percentage of CHF/COPD patients with specified treatment decisions documented in their medical records.

Process Measure: The percentage of CHF/COPD patients each month who have a clinic visit with an entry on their medical records documenting ever having a discussion of advance care plans.

Adverse-Effect Measure: The percentage of patients who are upset at having these issues raised and who decline the offer to help make plans.

All improvement requires change, but not all changes lead to improvement.

Working on your measurement plan often teaches you a lot about your aim; at that point, go back and restate the aim so that the aim and measure match (and also end up reflecting what you and your team really want to do).

IDENTIFYING AND TESTING CHANGES

With your aim and measures stated, your team needs to decide which changes to try. Of course, some interventions that you think will work may surprise you and behave otherwise. (That is why we test!) And remember that it is generally risky to implement a good idea on a large scale until you have it working well in one area with a few patients and staff.

How Do You Identify Which Changes to Make?

- Look at best practices
- Brainstorm ideas with your team
- Check the proven changes we recommend in this guide
- Keep a list of what has been tried and what is awaiting trial
- Select the changes that you are willing to try right away
- Be sure that the changes you try would make a difference in your measure and help accomplish your aim

Do's and Don'ts

- Do start with changes that you can do
  Do test the idea on a small scale to see if it works
- Don't do all the work yourself; delegate to the team and to others
- Do break down the work into smaller steps to make it less overwhelming
- Don't spend so much time preparing for a large-scale change that you don't get started quickly (say, by next Tuesday)

Good ideas are found everywhere; the challenge is to select the ones that are most worthwhile for you to try in your organization.

How Will I Know If an Idea Will Work for My System?

Once you have identified changes to try, assess them on a small sample of patients, clients, or nursing home residents. Testing is a step-by-step process to help identify whether or not something is working. If the change does not have a good effect on your outcome, testing will give you some ideas on how to adjust it or whether to try something else. The four steps outlined below are the heart of the rapid-cycle QI model.

STEP 1: PLAN By now, you have a change you would like to try. You have to plan for the test, so consider the following:

- Decide with your team how you will implement this change on a small scale (plan it step by step).
- Identify who will do what and when they will accomplish the task.
- Make some predictions about what you expect to happen after the change is implemented.
- Set deadlines for key steps.
- Identify the data you will need to see what effect this change has made during the test period.

STEP 2: DO After you have planned your change, try it. Be sure to do the following:

- Document problems and unexpected observations.
- Collect and monitor the data.

STEP 3: STUDY After implementing the change and collecting the data, get together with your team to analyze what happened, look at what the data say about the change, and summarize what you have learned from this test. Did your data and observations match what you had predicted for this change? If yes, what else happened? If not, then why not? Even failed tests teach teams a great deal about their care system.

STEP 4: ACT By now, you will know whether the change you tested is working. If it is, you can plan to implement it on a larger scale (e.g., with more patients or in another setting). However, if you find that the change did not work well on the small group, the team needs to evaluate what happened so as to get ideas on how to modify the change or whether to try something else. Either way, the cycle moves back to step one.

Keep trying until you find what works in your system. Generally, try many small changes, one at a time, rather than gambling on one large change. Let your mantra be: "We are going to give it a try; if it does not work, we will learn something from it."

 Remember: Measurement tells you what works and what does not.

Matching Aims, Measures, and Changes

You may find it surprisingly difficult to get an aim, a measure, and a change to fit together. It is important to work on this until it is right. A frequent error is mistaking a change for an aim. For example, a team might say their aim is that "within one month, every patient will have an assessment for symptoms within four hours of admission." At first, that sounds like a worthy aim, but it has a serious flaw: you do not actually care about this aim. The reason to want to assess symptoms is so that you can relieve them. That is the real aim. Doing the assessment quickly is an important change, one that might allow you to achieve the aim of having patients be comfortable, quickly; but it would not accomplish that on its own. So, incorporate the real goal of comfort into the team's aim statement, and make the changes serve that aim. Sometimes, the change is so closely tied to the aim that it hardly matters; but usually, using a change as the aim will be misleading down the road when you have accomplished the change, but the real goal has not been reached.

Usually, you can see the real aim by asking whether you would be satisfied achieving the aim and nothing else. If you had many assessments but no change in symptoms, you would not have succeeded in increasing the patient's comfort, so assessments alone are not the aim.

Usually, you will have one or two measures that directly track the aim, but you may also have a few others that track the changes (process measures). How good do your measures need to be? Certainly, they do not have to be perfect. If you have 10 units of effort to put into improvement, save one or two for measurement. Too much measurement will make you focus only on data collection, but too little will leave you without insight. The right amount of measurement is what it will take to convince a benevolent skeptic. This standard of the benevolent skeptic usually calls to mind some organizational leader you will have to convince, and that is fine. You will often find that you are your own most critical skeptic, so be benevolent.

Displaying the Data

There are two ways that many teams use to display their data, both to gain insight and to tell their stories: time series graphs and storyboards/poster boards:

Time Series Graphs

A well-run QI project must determine whether the changes tested resulted in improvement. The best way to do that is usually by collecting and plotting data over time. Figure 2.1 (called a *time series* or *run chart*) shows changes in a rate or tally (y-axis) over time (x-axis). Figure 2.2 displays a useful time-series chart.

Storyboards

A storyboard helps you to display your project to others in the organization. The storyboard helps the team to understand its own progress, and it can also be dramatically effective for showing your results to senior leaders, other staff, other organizations, patients and families,

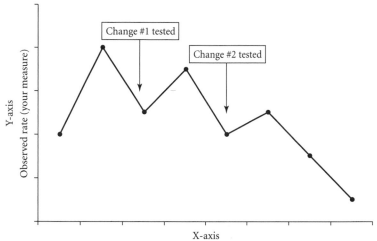

FIGURE 2.1 Annotated time series chart. Note the changes directly on your graph. This will help you identify the changes that made the greatest difference.

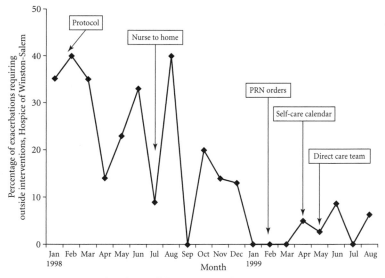

FIGURE 2.2 Example of a useful time series chart

policymakers, and the media. The storyboard should generally include the following:

1. Team information (including the names of team members and some contact information).
2. Brief description of the problem and the aim statement.
3. Brief description of your measures.
4. Time series graphs (to show your progress over time).
5. Successful changes that you have tried.
6. Challenges and lessons learned.
7. Other tools and resources that people might find helpful.

A storyboard can be printed and posted on a display board to show off at meetings and conferences. You can also post it in your work area, where team members can see it (an incentive to keep enthusiasm going). Other staff and family members may see the storyboard and encourage you or perhaps give you ideas about other strategies that might work. Posting the storyboard in your facility also gives the administrators a little reminder of your accomplishments every time they pass by. This will make your life easier when you find that you really need a few more nursing hours each week or a consultant to help manage pain for patients with complex needs.

Making the Changes Stick

After successfully implementing changes on a small scale, the challenge is to make them stick, so that old practices do not take over. Here are a few ideas on how to do this.

1. Establish and document the improved processes: procedures, guidelines, order sheets, forms, and so forth.
2. Revise job descriptions to make sure that someone is responsible for the new processes.

Creating a
Time Series

Do the Math

Most time series charts are a simple way to show *changes* over time. Plot weeks or months on the x-axis and the number or percentage of patients (or whatever you are measuring) on the y-axis. In the example below, the team tracked the percentage of exacerbations that required outside intervention and plotted it on the y-axis. The x-axis simply gives the month.

Is It Better to Track Number or Percentage?

If your denominator varies a good deal (e.g., one month you have 20 patients and the next month, 40), percentages give the most accurate picture of change over time. For example, suppose you are testing advance care plan documentation. In Month One, 20 out of 40 patients completed plans; in Month Two, 25 out of 75 patients complete plans. By the numbers, this would seem to show a slight improvement—but the percentages would show otherwise.

Usually the rate is the more informative figure, but it helps to keep the population size visible, for example 50% (of 40) or 33% (of 75). Sometimes, though, a tally is fine, especially when you are getting closer to ideal and tally any that fall short (e.g.,the number of transfers each month without advance care plans).

How Do I Get a Percentage for My Measurement?

You need two numbers to come up with the percentage: numerator and denominator.

$$\text{Percentage} = \frac{\text{Numerator (\# successful)}}{\text{Denominator (Total \# that have target characteristics)}} \times 100.$$

The numerator is the actual number that you have counted that shows your result, (e.g., the number of patients who have advance directives in their charts).

The denominator is the total number of patients who are in the population for whom you are implementing this change.

How Do I Create a Time Series?

You can use Excel to create time series graphs. However, you do not need to be technically savvy; you can create a time series graph using paper and pencil.

How to Annotate a Time Series Chart

Annotation means adding text information in your chart that tells you when you tried each intervention. This will help you in understanding which change made the most difference in getting your results. You should annotate the chart by adding text in text boxes in the chart (see the example of a time series chart).

3. Assign responsibility to particular people to monitor repeated backsliding (e.g., to report at staff meetings every quarter).
4. Add the new processes to training materials for new staff.
5. Tell others in your organization and community about your progress, and make participants proud of it. Share positive feedback from patients and families.

GIVE THEM SOMETHING TO TALK ABOUT

Once you have made improvements, spread the good word to other units in your organization or to other organizations. You can help to spread improvement by taking the following steps:

- Make the case for change by posting storyboards that show your success, by presenting your work in meetings or at conferences, and writing about your work in newsletters.
- Make it easier for others to do the work by thinking of your procedures, forms, and protocols as a kit that someone else could quickly put to use.
- Develop the messengers by supporting team members who are good communicators, helping them package the message, and finding forums in which to share it.

Early on in your project, think about ways to spread the improvement, and plan for how you will do so. Keep in mind the opportunities and barriers that you will face, and decide on a strategy that can get the most done within the limits of personnel and time. Hammer out these three following issues with your team:

Spread what: What will we have that could be worth implementing elsewhere?

Spread where: Who would benefit most from our work? Is it another kind of patient or another part of our organization?

Spread when: At what point in your project should you begin sharing it with others in your organization? When do you know your changes are really improvements, and how will you decide that your ideas are worth trying elsewhere?

Based on your answers, you can now develop an implementation plan to spread your process improvement.

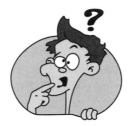

How to Motivate People
to Take on the Process
of Change Themselves

- Show evidence.
- Describe the benefits, tell patients' stories.
- Use your annotated time series to "tell the story."
- Target influential people and sites.
- Do not try to convince the most resistant people first.
- Build enthusiasm and commitment where you can.

FINAL RULES OF THUMB

It seems like a lot to keep in mind while trying to manage your "day job," too. Here are a few basic pointers to encourage you along the way.

- What can we do by next Tuesday? Keep it simple, and get it started.
- Set stretch goals that will make it worthwhile.
- Go for the low-hanging fruit by starting with easier projects or in units where staff will be friendly.
- You can only fix what you can measure.
- If we keep doing what we have been doing, we will keep getting what we have been getting. To get something better, we have to start doing something differently.

3

Advance Care Planning

In This Chapter

- Making timely care plans with patients and families
- Encouraging conversations among patients and loved ones
- Educating and involving clinicians
- Making decisions known and ensuring that they are followed

Many factors influence treatment decisions near the end of life: How old is the patient? How sick? Will treatment enhance life or mostly prolong suffering? What does the patient want? What does the family want? In the best-case scenario, the patient, family, and healthcare providers have discussed treatment options and preferences and documented these wishes in the form of an *advance care plan*. This way, everyone is prepared for eventual crises because they have agreed on a clear care plan that reflects the patient's values.

Although the issue has been increasingly in the public eye, few patients have had these discussions with their physician or family; and, even when they have, decisions may not be documented in the patient's record. Without plans, a crisis situation can escalate quickly, especially if the patient cannot communicate or if the family's preferences conflict with the clinician's. In these cases, treatment decisions are not made, they simply happen, usually based on habits that are presumed to reflect what patients generally want.

Decisions about naming a proxy decision-maker or about future care can be documented in legally authorized *advance directives* (ADs), such as *living wills,* or *durable powers of attorney for health care* (DPOAHC). ADs, however, are only one component of a more comprehensive approach called *advance care planning* (ACP). ACP results from a continuing dialogue between the patient, family, and healthcare providers, aiming to tailor clinical care to the patient's preferences and values, as well as to his or her clinical situation.

ACP can be challenging for the following reasons:

- Everyone is reluctant to talk about the patient's declining health and approaching death.
- Clinicians find it easier to offer comfort, hope, and medical technology rather than to "let people die."
- Patients and families find it hard to believe that treatments such as resuscitation will not restore health.
- Clinicians and family may not accept the patient's treatment priorities and values.

This chapter will help you meet these challenges by describing quality improvement (QI) projects that work. The story of Team Delta's project to improve ACP is based on a composite of several successful teams.

Team Delta

Team Delta is in a long-term care facility in a major city. About 20% of residents died each year. The facility had many ongoing QI programs, but nothing aimed at medical decision-making at the end of life. Team members had seen too many dying patients whose families insisted on tube feeding and hydration, even when doctors explained why these treatments would not be beneficial. Family members and staff agonized over what to do, especially when the resident could not communicate.

Families and physicians were left trying to puzzle out what would be best. The team wanted a better way to prepare patient, families, and staff for these situations. They wanted to try a more organized approach to medical decision-making and ACP, including ways to update records as treatment preferences changed.

Identifying the Problem and Setting an Aim

You may know that most of your seriously ill patients do not have good ACP, but you are not exactly sure where to start an improvement project. Do families always just want "everything done?" Are staff "afraid" to have these conversations earlier in the resident's stay because they "don't know what to say" or are afraid that they might "upset" the resident or family? Do patients really want to avoid these discussions? Before you act on your hunches, be sure that you know the problem well. Others on your team need to agree about what the problem really is. Your team might ask staff about their perceptions or ask residents' survivors. Do you have data that can clarify which are the most important areas or resident populations to start with? Even asking a few of your team members such questions can help identify the problem.

Team Delta

After a few brainstorming sessions, Team Delta talked to a few family members whose loved ones had recently been hospitalized or had died in the facility. They identified the following problem areas:

- *Residents, family, and staff were not aware of the need for ACP or the content of ACP discussions.*
- *Even residents at risk of dying did not routinely have a current ACP documented in their medical record, nor were they invited to participate in ACP discussions.*

- *For residents who had ACP discussions, completed ACPs often were not documented.*

Once Team Delta identified key problem areas, the team needed to set one or more aim statements that it could measure and toward which it could work. Team Delta developed the following aim statements to reflect its broad sequential goals:

Aim 1: *Within six months, 80% of the facility's professional caregivers will have participated in an educational seminar on ACP, treatment choices, and disease progression.*

Aim 2: *Within three months, 95% of new and "at risk of death" residents will have an ACP discussion documented in their medical records.*

Aim 3: *Within six months, 95% of new and "at risk of death" residents who have had an ACP discussion will have a completed advance care plan documented in their charts.*

The team then came up with this overarching aim statement.

Aim statement: *Within six months, 90% of new and "at risk of death" residents will have a completed ACP documented in their record (95% with discussion, and 95% of those discussions documented = 90% overall completion rate).*

What will improve: *Documented ACPs.*
By when: *Within six months.*
By how much: *Ninety percent (instead of the current occasional).*
For whom: *New and "at risk of death" residents.*

How to have comprehensive discussions with patients and families, how to document the patients' decisions and later changes in those decisions, and how to transfer patients' information to other healthcare settings are all part of a good ACP program. Common problems related to ACP include the following:

- Patients who are vulnerable and close to death end up getting inappropriate and undesired aggressive treatment because there is no other plan.
- Your healthcare system claims that ACPs are a priority, but no one knows how they are tracked, who is responsible for having them completed, or what is included in the discussions.
- Your practices encourage legal forms for advance directives but not more comprehensive and useful care planning.
- Your system documents many patients' decisions, but the care plan does not travel with the patients when they transfer to another unit or facility.
- Your protocol uses only a checklist of yes or no questions around the use of advanced technology with little regard for the social, psychological, or spiritual aspects of care planning.
- Your organization wants to make ACP a routine part of care, but only for patients very near death.
- Providers are reluctant to bring up ACP because they do not feel confident that they will know what to say or how to respond.

CHOOSING A TEAM

You have already identified the problem and created an aim statement. Now you need to invite other people who can help you reach your goals to join your team. Together, identify opportunities for improvement. For each patient population, try to recruit clinicians and others who are closest to them, such as physicians, nurses, social workers, and chaplains. Think beyond the obvious people, however, and you will discover others who can help make your program work. An admissions clerk, for instance, can help some projects by asking patients about whether they have an advance directive and where it is filed. If community adoption of a routine ACP process is part of the goal, your team can enlist colleagues who work in other settings to assist with procedures that assure that ACPs transfer with the patient or to recruit key players in your community.

Team Delta

The original force behind Team Delta was a unit nurse who had experienced too many overwhelmed families faced with complex medical treatment decisions for loved ones who were near death and could not communicate. She recruited a few of her coworkers, including a social worker, and sought advice and ideas from the facility's medical director. In order to raise awareness of the problem, Team Delta decided to focus on the team leader's unit as a starting point and involve the rest of the facility over time. In addition, they focused on new admissions, unstable patients, and severely demented residents as the first set of residents (and their families) to target. The team quickly realized that they would need help from a number of others in the facility, including the director of nursing, the staff educator, certified nursing assistants (CNAs) on the floor, and families. In addition, they would need help from the information specialists to flag charts electronically and to help measure their progress.

Measuring Success

Team Delta

To get a baseline, Team Delta reviewed 10 charts for residents who had died recently. No discussion of prognosis or treatment preferences had been documented, and no decisions had been made regarding life-sustaining treatments. Moreover, of the 10, six had died after being transferred to the hospital. The team decided to set a standard of having started a discussion with a resident and/or family member and documented existing decisions in the medical record within 72 hours of admission. The team started identifying "at risk of death" patients and severely cognitively impaired residents. Based on their aims, team members identified which measures they needed to track to best monitor their progress. Over the next few weeks, the team began to implement its changes, tracking whether the patient and family engaged in ACP; educating the facility staff on ACP and documentation of patient wishes; and assuring that their decisions were recorded.

Following are some of the measures other teams have tracked to follow their progress in ACP. The measures may be actual numbers or percentages. Your percentages must have a denominator (e.g., patients eligible for ACP) and a numerator (e.g., patients who complete advance directives). See Chapter 2 for more details.

Process Measures

- New admissions or targeted patients on a unit or floor who have an advance directive (AD) (e.g., DNR, healthcare proxy, living will).
- Providers using checklists of ACP topics and a "script" for discussions with patients.
- Patients and/or family caregivers who have completed an educational session on ACP.
- Healthcare providers can quickly find the patient's ACP.
- Targeted patients who have discussions with an ACP "SWAT" team within 48 hours of admission.

Outcome Measures

- Targeted patients who had an ACP discussion and decisions documented in their medical record within 48 hours of admission.
- Targeted patients whose documented treatment decisions were followed during serious illness.

- New admissions or targeted patients with discussions of ACP.
- Families saying that the discussion and decision-making were helpful or very helpful.

Adverse-Effect Measures

- Family members of patients who complain about the "focus on things going badly."
- Family members who say that ACP discussions are "too formal" or "too impersonal."
- Families who have some family members disagree with the patient's AD.
- Patients who insist upon a generally unwise course of care, rather than opting for a trial of treatment or allowing for later decisions by a proxy.

TELLING YOUR STORY: TIME SERIES CHARTS

Time series charts are an effective way to quickly tell the story of your results. Below are two of Team Delta's time series charts. The changes they tested are noted on the following graphs and explained below.

IDENTIFY AND TEST CHANGES

Once Team Delta finalized its aims and how to track them, it looked at best practices to identify good ideas to try on the study unit.

TEAM DELTA

The team decided to try the following ideas:

1. *Invite residents and families to attend a class that provides information on various options and helps them to complete ACP forms.*

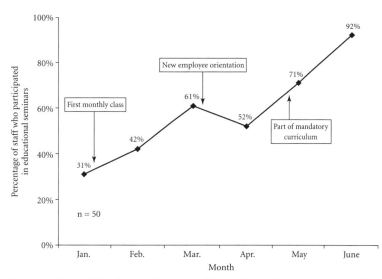

FIGURE 3.1 Within six months, 80% of the facility's direct caregivers will have participated in an educational seminar on advance care planning, treatment choices, and disease progression.

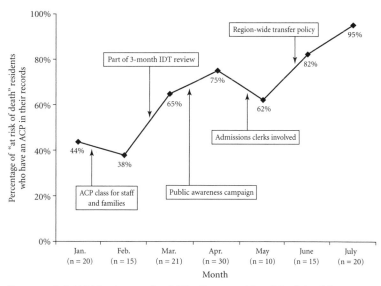

FIGURE 3.2 Within six months, 90% of new and "at risk of death" residents will have a completed advance care plan documented.

2. *Offer mandatory classes for clinicians to help them understand and initiate ACP discussions, including role playing.*
3. *Involve frontline staff, such as admissions clerks, to get the advance directive forms completed and entered into the system.*
4. *Develop a staff education and public awareness campaign within the facility to raise awareness, understanding, and recognition of the importance of ACP.*
5. *Make ACP review part of the routine quarterly interdisciplinary team (IDT) meetings.*
6. *Reach out to hospital partners to settle on standardized and adequate documentation and "transfer" procedures for ACP.*

With the help and dedication of team members, Team Delta tried one change at a time. Once a strategy showed better results, they implemented it on a larger scale.

There are a number of ways that you can improve ACP for your patients. Here are some interventions that QI teams have tried and that have proven successful:

Change Ideas to Improve ACP

- Develop a systematic approach and designate providers to initiate, document, and complete ACPs (e.g., list of topics to cover, who is responsible for each item, where the documents will be kept, etc.).
- Add a pop-up box about ACP availability on the computer order screen (e.g., when DNR order is written, at admission, or at discharge from the hospital).
- Conduct automatic ACP review at quarterly IDT conferences in long-term care institutions.
- Incorporate questions about proxy and DNR orders into admission forms with more comprehensive follow-up by

clinicians (e.g., ACP "SWAT" team) while in the hospital or nursing home.

- Encourage time-limited trials for invasive technology or treatments with agreement about when to stop.
- Be clear about DNR and proxy orders at admission; use community follow-up (with primary-care physicians, community social workers, home health providers, and other providers in the system) to continue and complete ACP documents and periodically review them with patient and family.
- Standardize ACP procedures, to be completed in a set time frame (e.g., 72 hours after admission; within one week of admission; etc.).
- Develop standardized "scripts" for starting ACP discussions. One of the best openings: "At this time in your life, what is it that makes you happy?" Then, ask the same question regarding what makes you "sad" or "anxious." Then discuss prognosis and other difficult issues (see Physician Orders for Life-Sustaining Treatment (POLST) in the Resources section at the end of this chapter).
- Implement a standardized healthcare proxy form for use throughout the institution.
- Train clinicians to conduct family meetings, help patients and families to express wishes and make decisions, and document the settled plan of care.
- Develop posters, brochures, and similar material for patients and family members. For example, staff can wear buttons that ask, "I Have an Advance Care Plan, Do You?" or "Ask Me about Advance Care Planning."
- Monitor the process of ACP and patient and family reaction to it, as well as the accuracy of documentation of patient wishes on transfer.
- Make plans about the patient's preferred place to die.

As you think about changes you would like to make, plan for obstacles. QI teams frequently encounter similar barriers, regardless of the setting in which they are working. Below is a list of common barriers; remember that others have overcome them—and you can, too:

Common Barriers to ACP

- Not being able to offer key treatment options, such as palliative sedation or clinician visits in the home for symptom exacerbation, really limits how much you can improve things for your patients.
- "The big lie" that all will be well and that we do not need to deal with this. For example, during inpatient rehabilitation for older people, it is tempting to communicate a sense that the patient is not really up against a serious, chronic condition but is just a little off course and on the verge of recovery. That lie means not only that death comes as a shock to family but also that no useful care planning can take place.
- Patients may express a desire to die at home, but the caregiver may fear being unable to manage worsening health at home. In this case, you need to think about what you can really offer in terms of support (on-call physicians, hospice, oxygen, etc.) and what the family can manage.
- Multiple physicians and other providers, with no real communication among them, leave the patient and family with the sense that no one is in charge or responsible, that no one grasps the situation accurately, and that no one can really ensure that the ACP is followed.
- Providers may be reluctant to "bring up bad news" (e.g., they may be uncomfortable with the conversation, they do not

know how to start such a talk, etc.). In this case, groups find that providing physicians and nurses with a script to follow helps them overcome their anxieties.

- Providers fear that patients do not want to have these discussions.

GIVE THEM SOMETHING TO TALK ABOUT

To give them something to talk about, get started. Here are a few key points to remember:

1. Get started on the project, and do not wait for everything to be perfect.
2. Do not carry a lot of baggage from limited interpretations of your state's laws. This may require challenging overly restrictive institutional procedures.
3. Get feedback from patients and families to find out how you are doing and to get the boost that you may need to continue your efforts.
4. Do not just focus on CPR; instead, build ACP discussions around a good life, right up to the end.
5. Address the practical issues that your patients face, such as whom to call in time of need, which medication to take, and how symptoms will progress.
6. Use every crisis situation survived as an opportunity for rehearsing preferred options. Ask the patient and family (and professional care givers) what should have been done, and what can be done differently next time.
7. Avoid using medical jargon. Tailor your language to your setting and patients. "Artificial hydration" may not mean much to a 75-year-old spouse.

FREQUENTLY ASKED QUESTIONS

What Should We Discuss When Deciding ACPs?

- Present the clinical situation, now and in the future, and options for the care plan in more than one way so as to ensure comprehension.
- Discuss the patient's health status and quality of life following treatment.
- When using medical technology, offer the use of time-limited trials rather than forcing a choice between "never" and "forever."
- Promise reassessment on a scheduled basis, and promise to stop if treatment is not helping.
- Listen to the patient, allowing time for him or her to respond and express wishes, fears, and concerns.
- Honor the search for meaning, treat symptoms, and ensure continuity.
- Set reasonable expectations for prognosis and treatments: what can your system promise the patient in the last years and weeks of life.
- Support families through all phases of illness, and plan for bereavement issues after death.
- Be capable of and willing to provide sedation for those near death if that is what the patient needs.

What Are Some of the Communication Strategies Needed to Initiate ACPs?

Some useful communication strategies are summarized for you in Table 3.1 on pages 57–59.

Table 3.1 What Are Some of the Communication Strategies to Initiate Advance Care Planning (ACP)?

Health Status	Content of Discussions	Action Items	Suggested Communication Strategy
Healthy people	▪ Identification and notification of surrogate/proxy decision-maker. ▪ Identification of preferences about undesirable outcome states (e.g., persistent vegetative state). ▪ Note atypical beliefs or preferences (e.g., Jehovah's Witness).	▪ May complete durable power of attorney. ▪ Discuss proxy appointment and values with surrogate. ▪ Write down preferences.	▪ "There are many drugs that we can use to treat your hypertension; one is less expensive, but you must take it twice a day. A second must be taken only once a day, but it costs more." ▪ "If you become too sick to speak with me about your healthcare preferences, with whom would you want me to speak?" ▪ "Do you have any specific concerns that you would like to share with me?" ▪ "In some states, your preference to forgo a feeding tube if you are terminally ill or in a prolonged coma is only honored if it is written down in your advance directive."

(continued)

Table 3.1 (continued)

Health Status	Content of Discussions	Action Items	Suggested Communication Strategy
Diagnosed with a serious illness	• Same as above. • What is important for you now (values, beliefs, psychosocial needs)? • Discuss treatment burden and potential adverse-outcome states. • Discuss time-limited trials of treatments (not "never vs. always"). • Discuss likely course with proposed treatments and likely outcomes. • Discuss what the next steps could be in the follow-up and management of the patient's condition.	• Same as above. • MD discusses prognoses and Outcomes, with and without recommended treatments • MD/RN talks to surrogate. • MD/RN offers spiritual support.	• "I anticipate that you will have a good recovery from this stroke. We are going to treat you with a blood thinner that will substantially reduce your risk of a further stroke. However, the risk is not zero. It is important to plan ahead. Do you have any concerns or thoughts about your medical care if you do not have a good recovery?" • "Unlike TV shows, resuscitation is rarely effective when your mother has a serious illness like a stroke that produces unconsciousness." • "What do you know about what is likely to happen?

Diagnosed with serious illness that will limit life expectancy, or coming to the end of a long life.	▪ Same as above. ▪ Explicit discussion about courses of potential treatments, likely outcomes, individual economic consequences. ▪ Discussion of time-limited trials of treatments. ▪ What is important for you to accomplish in the time you have left? ▪ How can I help you achieve this?	▪ Same as above. ▪ State specific preferences and formulate contingency plans. ▪ Be sure that key decisions are written down and transferred with the patient.	▪ "Mrs. X, your breathing is really a problem for you almost all of the time now. Tell me a little about your thoughts. In this part of your life, what makes you truly happy? What makes you worried or upset? What do you think will happen? What do you hope for? What do you hope to avoid? What do you expect the end to be like?" ▪ "You said that you want medical care to focus on comfort. Even if you get more short of breath, you want to stay home. Is that correct? If you do get short of breath, and it does not respond to usual treatments, we will use morphine and your family can call. . . ."

Tools and Resources

- Handbook for Mortals
  http://www.medicaring.org
- Caring Connections
  http://www.caringinfo.org
- POLST
  http://www.ohsu.edu/ethics/polst/
- Respecting Choice Program, Gunderson Lutheran, La Crosse, Wisconsin
  http://www.gundluth.org/eolprograms
- Five Wishes
  http://www.agingwithdignity.org/
- Vermont Ethics Network
  http://www.vtethicsnetwork.org/
- Gold Standard Framework for Palliative Care
  http://www.goldstandardsframework.nhs.uk/

4

Preventing, Assessing, and Treating Pain

In This Chapter

- Defining pain
- Making pain the "Fifth Vital Sign"
- Using clinical practice guidelines
- Setting standards for pain control
- Reviewing prescribing practices

Severe pain in a dying person is unacceptable, and its consequences are severe: Inadequate pain relief can hasten death, lead to despair, and destroy the patient's quality of life.

Despite advances in pain management, many barriers still prevent people from receiving effective treatment. In some cases, patients may be reluctant to talk about their pain, fearing that they will seem weak or that they will become dependent on pain medicine. Sometimes, it can take hours (in hospitals) or even days (in home care) to get pain medicine to a patient, once it has been ordered.

A few basic steps can improve pain management. Doctors and nurses need to talk to patients about pain; they should ask about comfort (usual, worst, what helps, how it affects the patient), discuss treatment options, and provide information about the nature of pain and how to control it. Knowing that their healthcare team is listening and that everyone involved is confident that pain can be managed can comfort patients and their families.

The case study throughout this chapter represents a composite of work done by various successful teams with which we have worked. Their efforts illustrate how a team can identify a problem, come up with an aim, and measure the results of the changes it has made (see Chapter 2 for basic methods).

TEAM FAITH

Some oncology nurses in Faith Hospice realized that cancer patients were often in pain, despite efforts by medical and nursing staff to relieve it. The nurses wanted to do something about it—but what? Should they identify specific problems in the hospice program, or should they jump right in with ideas that they think will fix things? Should they recruit other people to be on their team? What should Team Faith do?

Even when doctors and nurses assess pain, they may have neither sufficient resources to treat and manage it, nor the staffing resources to reassess and monitor pain levels. Teams need to realize their limitations and have expert referrals and backup available.

IDENTIFYING THE PROBLEM AND SETTING AN AIM

Like Team Faith, you may know that patients are in pain but not know which ones are most likely to suffer and why. If your care setting is like others nationwide, chances are that your patients with advanced cancer are in pain. According to one report, almost 75% of advanced cancer patients admitted to the hospital report being in pain upon admission. Even for those known to be very near the end of life, those in pain number more than half of the admissions. What is it about current pain management protocols that is not working, and can you fix it? Nationally, women, older adults, and minorities are most likely to be under-treated for pain; what is your situation? You will need to characterize areas in which you are falling short in order to see how you might improve.

Start by forming a team of concerned and involved staff. Together, characterize why patients are in pain despite your current efforts. Discuss some examples (review four or five charts) and figure out the patterns.

Once you have settled on an aim, decide how to measure a trend toward success. Does the patient's pain rating decrease with each shift? Do other quality-of-life indicators improve? Is the patient better able to function? Is the pain level always below the patient's goal?

TEAM FAITH

Rather than acting on vague ideas about a few cases, Team Faith met to discuss what each member observed, what existing data showed, and what to do. They talked about possible changes and how to test them. After a few meetings, the team chose the following aim, one around which the whole team could rally.

Aim: By August, 95% of cancer patients admitted to our hospice program will never again have pain that is worse than their pain goal and which lasts for more than eight hours.

What will improve: Pain will always be below each patient's personal pain goal within eight hours.
By when: August.
By how much: For 95% of all enrolled patients.
For whom: Cancer patients admitted to hospice with pain as a problem.

CHOOSING A TEAM

To succeed, your team must include the key players from your organization and community. Selecting the team takes thinking through the process needed to achieve your aim. Include the admissions nurse if early identification is a big issue, or involve the pharmacy delivery runner if slow response time is a target. Try to include at least these three: an administrator who will champion your cause; someone who knows quality improvement (QI) methods, and someone who knows a lot about pain prevention and treatment.

TEAM FAITH

Once the three hospice nurses decided to test changes to improve pain relief for cancer patients, they needed to add key people to their team. Eventually, Team Faith included a pharmacist, an oncologist, a palliative care nurse, and the hospital's vice president for patient services. In addition, one of the nurses had training in QI methods.

MEASURING SUCCESS

Whatever your aim, three basic measures can be used in the rapid-cycle process: outcome, process, and adverse effects (also see Chapter 2). For example, Team Faith's outcome measures included pain levels below the patient's own target. For you, process measures might include routine assessment or rapid response time. And adverse-effect measures should be monitored for trouble that stems from your changes (e.g., constipation or delirium).

Decide which data to collect, who will collect it and when, and how and whether to sample the population. Depending on the number of patients with which you are dealing, you may not have enough time to look at every record or patient. Instead, you will need a sampling plan. You also need to decide how often to display your data: weekly, monthly, or quarterly. Be sure to collect enough data to build a case (or to monitor when an improvement is not working).

TEAM FAITH

Once Team Faith had invited key players to join them and had agreed on an aim, they worked out the specifics of how to measure whether their efforts were making a difference.

Measure: Percentage of cancer patients admitted to hospice with pain on their health problem list, who live the rest of their lives with no period longer than eight hours with pain worse than their personal goal.

If you look closely at Team Faith's aim statement, the measure is closely linked to the aim (see above).

Take note of the following specific reasons that are the basis of the aim:

- Some "successful" patients will never have serious pain, while others will have serious pain for less than eight hours. This is a compromise to simplify data collection and evaluation.
- Why lifelong? Because this team had an electronic record system that could readily search for pain worse than personal level and test for relief within eight hours. Cancer patients in hospice overwhelmingly stay in the program until death.
- Why less than patient goal? Some teams might choose an amount less than four (on a 0–10 scale). The standard this team chose is closest to what matters to patients, yet it does require collaborating with patients to establish their pain goal and getting it recorded in the electronic record.
- Why 95% and not 100%? The team knew at the start that the rate was running no better than 50%, so 95% was quite a change. But they also knew that some patients just could not give up their pain for all sorts of reasons, so they did not believe that the "best care" would be 100%.

- Why eight hours? The nurses felt that a 95% success rate would require that most patients were brought under control within a few hours, but they were also aware that no one would want to have to wake up a patient or family member just to confirm success. Also, some situations require trying a few strategies. The team considered 24 hours but rejected that as not being good enough for a promise to patients and families.

Sometimes, collecting data on outcome measures alone is not enough, or it is not possible. You may need to look at the process itself and collect data to check that it is working.

TEAM FAITH

Team Faith decided to start off measuring one process and one adverse effect.

Process measure: Percentage of cancer patients with the patient's target level and their current level of pain recorded with initial vital signs.

Adverse-effect measure: Percentage of cancer patients with opioid medications for whom a successful bowel regimen is continued or a new or improved one started.

Pain improvement teams can choose from many outcomes to measure progress. The following ideas should inspire you to think about what is important in your environment:

- Increased patient confidence in pain relief (outcome).
- Improved pain documentation (process).
- Reduced waiting time for pain medications (process).
- Reduced pain (outcome).
- Eliminated use of meperidine for chronic pain (process).

- Reduced or eliminated errors in changing from one opioid to another (adverse effect).
- Nurse satisfaction with pain management (adverse effect).

Following are some sample measures for improving pain treatment:

Process Measures

- Pain documentation on 100% of admissions.
- Waiting time for inpatient pain medications reduced to less than one hour.
- Rapidly escalating dosage is recognized and leads to palliative care consultation and evaluation within eight hours.
- Eliminate the use of meperidine for chronic pain.

Outcome Measures

- Patient survey shows 90% confidence in pain relief.
- After patients' deaths, 85% of families state that there was never a time when pain was out of control.
- Pain of less than five (0–10 scale) within eight hours of pain complaint.

Adverse-Effect Measures

- Eliminate errors in changing from one opioid to another (measure the time between errors).
- Nurses report problems with pain management.

TELLING YOUR STORY: TIME SERIES CHART

TEAM FAITH

To measure its progress, Team Faith compiled data for a chart that showed what percentage of patients dying each month had achieved their own pain management goal each week. To measure improvement, the team used the electronic record to identify pain that was out of control and when it was reported. Then the system calculated whether relief was documented within eight hours.

For the numerator, Team Faith used the number of patients whose pain level was less than the patient's own preferred level at all times or within eight hours of reporting a pain problem. (These patients represent a subset of the denominator.)

The denominator was the total number of cancer patients in hospice who: (1) had any pain problem in their problem list; (2) were able to state their preferred level and their actual level; and (3) had died that month in hospice care.

The team tracked its results on the time series chart shown in Figure 4.1.

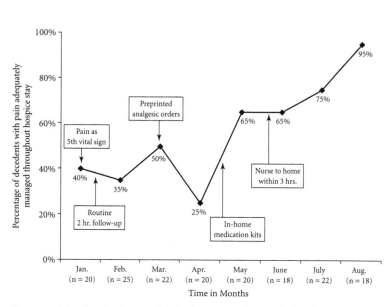

FIGURE 4.1 Aim: By August, 95% of cancer patients admitted to our hospice program will never again have pain worse than their pain goal lasting more than eight hours.

IDENTIFYING AND TESTING CHANGES

TEAM FAITH

To reach its aim, Team Faith eventually chose five changes.

1. *Make pain the "Fifth Vital Sign," which is recorded on admission and on every contact with patient or family.*
2. *Change the current pain protocol so that nurses routinely follow up with patients every two hours until the pain goal is met.*
3. *Involve physicians and pharmacists in developing preprinted order sets to get escalations of doses to patients promptly.*
4. *Have kits of backup medications in the home to cover the most likely escalation of the dose.*
5. *For severe pain, be able to have a nurse at the home within three hours.*

Team Faith made each change on a small scale by having one nurse try out the new processes on her patients. By testing one change at a time, the team could see which changes led to improvements. When they were satisfied that the change was working smoothly and improved performance, they included more nurses and patients. In the first few weeks, the team was disappointed to find that patient pain measurements were not improving. Team members spent time observing how the changes were being implemented, and they helped the frontline nurses change the workflow so that they had the scale at hand to help patients and families report on pain.

Other successful pain improvement teams have tried changes such as the following.

- Eliminate barriers to getting pain medication delivered to patients.
- Have a backup physician prescribe drugs if the attending physician is not available within a specific time.

- Educate patients, families, and healthcare providers about the nature of opioid analgesics and explain why they are not dangerous.
- Make a follow-up call to outpatients two days after discharge to assess the need for a medication change and to prescribe the change by phone.
- Post pain scales at each patient bedside.
- Give outpatients a pain diary to track pain and the effect of medications taken at home.
- Assess depression and anxiety, especially for patients with pain greater than level five (on a 0–10 scale, see below).

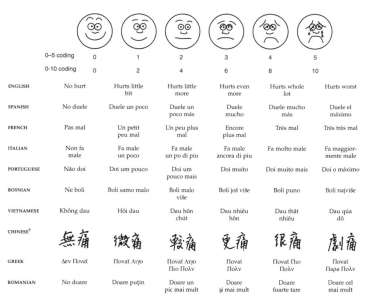

FIGURE 4.2 Wong-Baker FACES Pain Scale. From Hockenberry, J. J., Wilson, D., & Winkelstein, M. L. (2005). *Wong's Essentials of Pediatric Nursing* (7th ed., p. 1259). St. Louis: Elsevier. Used with permission.

- Some patients who have trouble rating pain on a 0–10 scale can use a FACES scale (see Figure 4.2).
- Distribute educational materials on pain treatment to patients so that they know what to expect.
- Give patients and families a "sure-fire" fallback plan, such as paging the covering physician or house supervisor nurse.

COMMON BARRIERS TO GOOD PAIN MANAGEMENT

All improvement efforts encounter barriers. Anticipating and preparing for them will allow your team to overcome problems while staying focused on your aim. Although the Joint Commission on Accreditation of Healthcare Organizations generally does not welcome standby kits at home, our teams have found them to be quite effective in helping patients and caregivers to manage at home. Of course, kits should be provided only after careful instruction and training on their use.

Common Barriers

- Inadequate knowledge of pain assessment, prevention, and treatment.
- Difficulty of measuring pain in nonverbal patients (but see the pain and dementia citation at the end of this chapter).
- Differing priorities of patients and their families regarding pain management.
- Concern about side effects of medication.
- Reluctance to take medications due to fear of addiction.
- The patient thinks that pain is an inevitable consequence of disease.
- Pain response is just not a high priority for staff in the hospital.

TEAM FAITH

Initially, Team Faith struggled to meet patients' pain goals. The team found that many patients were setting unrealistic goals, hoping for a pain level of zero when their condition would indicate that some discomfort would remain. Other patients refused to take medications, making pain management impossible. To counter this, Team Faith worked with nursing staff to address the challenge of patients who refused medication or who had set unrealistic pain levels. The team provided information about pain management to all patients and their families and wrote a script to help nurses manage conversations about pain control. Team Faith made sure that doctors talked to patients who had refused medications. Team Faith also found that drug delivery times were sometimes greater than eight hours, a finding that led to keeping standby kits in the home.

GIVE THEM SOMETHING TO TALK ABOUT

Pain management presents an area where improvement can have dramatic effects. Remember the following:

- Promise your patients comfort but explain that they are not likely to be completely pain-free.
- Prescribe opioids whenever needed, but monitor the effects.
- Empower patients and their families to manage pain by giving them a range of doses that are under their control.
- Do not use meperidine (which can cause seizures and hallucinations and often does not last long enough to control pain adequately).
- Have anesthetic and nonpharmacological approaches readily available.

- Watch for side effects of opioids, such as constipation.
- Assume that patients on pain medication will need adjustments. Follow up at appropriate intervals, both soon after change and in other regularly scheduled intervals.
- Make sure that the conversion of drugs and the mode of administration are done correctly.

TEAM FAITH

Once Team Faith met its goal, the team made sure that its progress did not slip. The team trained all current and new providers on the new processes. They also posted the new processes at every nursing workstation and on field notepads. They placed the new forms in an appropriate place so that everyone remembered to use them. With everyone's help, the team sustained the changes and made them permanent. Eventually, other healthcare professionals began to use the new approach, and it soon became part of a system-wide pain management initiative.

FREQUENTLY ASKED QUESTIONS

What Are Some Nonpharmacologic Ways to Treat Pain?

- Neurostimulation: Transcutaneous Electrical Nerve Stimulation (TENS), acupuncture.
- Anesthesiologic: nerve block.
- Physical therapy: exercise, heat, cold.
- Psychological approaches: cognitive therapies (relaxation, imagery, hypnosis).
- Biofeedback: behavior therapy, psychotherapy.
- Complementary therapies: massage, art, music, aromatherapy.
- Distraction.

What Are Some of the Common and Uncommon Side Effects of Opioids?

Common Side Effects

- Constipation
- Dry mouth
- Nausea/vomiting
- Sedation
- Sweats

Uncommon Side Effects

- Bad dreams/hallucinations
- Dysphoria/delirium
- Myoclonus/seizures
- Pruritus/urticaria
- Respiratory depression
- Urinary retention

What Are Some Changes to Try in Managing Pain and Other Symptoms?

- Widely accepted guidelines for cancer pain are followed.
- Low rate of orders for breakthrough pain (repeated need to treat breakthrough symptoms should trigger increased regular doses of pain medications).
- Rescue dose is always available.
- When pain is continuous, all opioids are on a regular dosing schedule.
- Patients and families control the timing of dosing for breakthrough pain.
- Sufficient pain medication is provided during medical procedures and transfers between units and facilities.

- On a 0–10 scale, pain greater than three requires intervention; pain greater than six is an emergency). Patient receives emergency response, then root-cause error analysis.
- Clinician performance is routinely reviewed, and shortcomings are addressed.
- Clinicians attend to and manage predictable side effects.
- Patients and families learn about pain management issues from clinicians and staff.
- Assess pain, depression, dyspnea, and anxiety on a specified schedule (e.g., admission, change in status, and periodically) 100% of the time.
- Use all appropriate modalities, often on time-limited trials, including opioids, non-steroidal anti-inflammatory drugs (NSAIDS), adjuvant analgesics, physical therapy (apply heat and cold), massage therapy, behavioral techniques, steroids, neuroablative procedures, stimulants, and so forth.
- Have skilled consultants readily available to patients in all settings (including ICU, hospital, nursing home, hospice, and home).
- During transfers between units or sites, prevent pain by holding the sending and receiving parties responsible for being sure that the patient is comfortable and relatively pain free.

TOOLS AND RESOURCES

What Are the Best Tools That I Can Use to Assess My Patients' Pain?

- Wong/Baker FACES Scale (detailed information on how to use the FACES Scale is available along with the downloads) http://www3.us.elsevierhealth.com/WOW/faces.html

- Pain Assessment in Advanced Dementia (PAINAD) (five-item observational tool for caregivers)
  http://mqa.dhs.state.tx.us/QMWeb/Pain/PAINAD.htm
- Edmonton Symptom Assessment System (ESAS) (tool to assess nine symptoms in cancer patients)
  http://www.palliative .org/PC/ClinicalInfo/AssessmentTools/
      esas.pdf
- Assessing Pain in Persons with Dementia
  http://www.hartfordign.org/publications/trythis/assessingPain
      .pdf

What Are Some Good Web Sites Where I Can Find Pain Resources?

- City of Hope Pain/Palliative Care Resource Center
  http://mayday.coh.org
- Beth Israel Medical Center, Department of Pain Medicine and Palliative Care
  http://www.stoppain.org/
- ICU Delirium and Cognitive Impairment Study Group: Brain Dysfunction in Critically Ill Patients
  http://www.icudelirium.org/delirium/
- National Center for Complementary and Alternative Medicine
  http://www.nccam.nih.gov

5

ASSURING COMFORT

IN THIS CHAPTER

- Identifying burdensome symptoms
- Understanding elements of good symptom management
- Using clinical practice guidelines and other resources
- Using quality improvement to ensure patient comfort

For patients, the experience of illness is often the long story of symptoms and associated suffering and fear. For clinicians, symptoms present diagnostic clues and therapeutic challenges. Controlling symptoms often defines good medical care, particularly for advanced and incurable illnesses, when the patient's priorities focus on comfort and quality of life. Although pain may be the most prominent symptom associated with advanced disease and the end of life, many other symptoms contribute to patient suffering, including dyspnea, fatigue, delirium, depression, anorexia, cachexia, hypoxia, nausea and vomiting, and constipation.

Good practice for symptom management is logical (even when our real-world approach is not).

- Know which symptoms are present by asking the patient (or family, if the patient cannot communicate).
- Ask whether anything has helped in the past. Find out what

the symptom means to the patient (e.g., is dyspnea terrifying or just exhausting? Is depression blocking the patient's ability to spend time with family?) Consider any alternative approaches that the patient has found worthwhile—for example, acupuncture or massage therapy—as they may be worth trying again.

- Look for the cause (or, at least, the likely cause) of the symptom.
- Know what works to relieve and prevent this symptom in similar cases, and work with patients and caregivers to make a plan.
- Try out the plan. If it works, great. If not, promptly try something else.
- Be sure to follow up since patients and families often think that they must live with even more severe symptoms.

Keep in mind the following key points for symptom management for end-of-life patients.

- Trust the patient's report of his or her experience. When patients cannot speak, you will have to decide which evidence to trust; just remember that the more common error is to underrecognize and undertreat symptoms.
- Consider all available treatments and their merits in the context of the patient's values, culture, goals, and fears.
- When illness is advanced, and death is near, the exact causes of any given symptom often become irrelevant, but the symptom still must be relieved.
- Anxiety, fatigue, and emotional and psychological stress worsen the experience of the symptoms (and vice versa).
- The psychological component of every symptom presents an opportunity to heal the psyche while relieving the symptoms.

This chapter will help you to improve symptom management in advanced illness and at the end of life. By following the basic quality improvement (QI) process described in Chapter 2, you too can develop a project that improves comfort. "Team Breathe-Easy" is a composite based on many groups that have successfully improved their symptom management practices.

TEAM BREATHE-EASY

Physicians and nurses from acute care, community palliative care, and the lung-disease clinic realized that their chronic obstructive pulmonary disease (COPD) patients were not doing well at managing their symptoms at home. Instead, they frequently appeared in the emergency room, frightened and overwhelmed by dyspnea, or they cancelled appointments, complaining that they were just too tired to move. These healthcare providers decided that together, they had to do something to help their patients. But what? The brochures and posters around the clinic were just not enough to help patients learn good self-management techniques. But what could these busy healthcare professionals do? And how? Should they collect data on a unit or jump right in with promising ideas? Should they recruit other people from various clinics to be on their team? What would you do?

IDENTIFYING THE PROBLEM AND SETTING AN AIM

The exact shape of your project will depend on your own situation and the problems that you identify. Because pain is one of the most common symptoms for advanced illness and at the end of life, many QI teams focus on relieving it. However, many other difficult symptoms, such as dyspnea or pressure ulcers, can be addressed using rapid-cycle QI. Here is a list of several target symptoms:

Common Symptoms

- Pain (see Chapter 4)
- Fatigue (asthenia)
- Anorexia (loss of appetite)
- Cachexia (loss of weight)
- Drowsiness or insomnia
- Confusion
- Anxiety
- Dyspnea (shortness of breath)
- Nausea and vomiting
- Constipation and diarrhea
- Delirium
- Depression

How to Identify Target Symptoms

- Which symptoms do your patients fear most?
- Which are most common?
- Which situations involving symptom management are most upsetting to your staff?
- Which problem areas are most readily solved?

After you have identified the symptoms that your system should improve, you should state your aim (see Chapter 2 for how to create an aim statement).

TEAM BREATHE-EASY

Team Breathe-Easy wanted to meet the physical, psychosocial, and spiritual needs of its COPD patients and families; but that was a tall order, and too general to use as an aim. Realizing that they did not know where to start, they contacted 12 patients who had been readmitted to the COPD unit within 60 days of discharge and asked them two questions: Why had they come to the hospital? Could anything have enabled them to deal with the issue at home? The responses confirmed what Team Breathe-Easy had suspected: Patients and caregivers were not confident that they could do anything to manage symptoms at home. The team decided to better support symptom management at home as a way to reduce the experience of dyspnea and hospital readmission rate. The team agreed on the following aim statement to achieve its goal.

Aim: *Within six months, 85% of advanced COPD patients discharged with comprehensive home-care services will be comfortable at home and will not be readmitted to the hospital within three months of discharge.*

What will improve: *Home-based symptom management, so that patients are comfortable at home and are not readmitted to hospital within three months of discharge.*
By when: *Within six months.*
By how much: *Eighty-five percent, rather than current rate of 50%.*
For whom: *Advanced COPD patients discharged with comprehensive home-care service.*

Choosing a Team

Based on your project's focus, try to include knowledgeable providers who can help patients and their families cope with the array of symptoms that people face at the end of life. To be manageable, your core group should include five to seven stakeholders, people who are really invested in your aim and project.

Our hospital-based teams often report that success usually hinges on a physician "champion" who can provide clinical expertise and a link to senior management. Your champion need not be a physician, but it should be someone who knows the field, who has the clinical and administrative authority to implement a QI project, and who is going to be around for a year (or more) to see the work through. Beyond this, your team should be made up of those who "own the process" and "make things happen." Your team could be enriched with input from many experts: a geriatric psychiatrist, a palliative care physician, a hospital pharmacist, a nutritionist or dietitian, or a family member would each be able to offer insights and suggestions that your team could use.

TEAM BREATHE-EASY

Team Breathe-Easy included two physicians and two nurses who had responsibilities in the hospital, home health care, and the COPD clinic. Once the core team had its aim, they sought support from others who worked with their patient population. Eventually, the team expanded to include a nurse from the community health program, a respiratory therapist, and a social worker. The group also turned to staff from the Ask-a-Nurse hotline, which served the entire suburban area, and others from pulmonary rehabilitation, smoking cessation, and the IT group. As its work progressed, the core team kept senior administrators posted on what was happening and what had yet to be done. A few months into their work, the team expanded to include a particularly engaged patient, a man who had been a construction engineer. His presence (while on oxygen) turned out to be quite motivating and kept the team focused on the patient perspective.

MEASURING SUCCESS

How do you turn abstract ideas into measurable aims? In rapid-cycle QI, three kinds of measures work best to track whether changes are actually improvements: process, outcome, and adverse effect.

We recommend that you choose one key measure to track your progress; once underway, consider adding one or two others. The nature of your project is likely to drive decisions about the type of data to collect. Your team needs to decide who will collect the data and when, as well as how to sample the data (see Chapter 2 for more details on measures). Depending on the number of patients you treat, you might not have enough time to get data about every patient. If so, you will want to pick a sample for your study. Team Breathe-Easy, for instance, might track everyone discharged in the first 10 days of each month. You might find that your baseline data can be obtained through the IT department and in records already maintained, such as hospitalization dates. In addition, your team will have to decide how frequently to collect data: daily, weekly, monthly, or quarterly.

Each QI team will develop its own measures—and may be surprised by how many ways it can track a project. The following process, outcome, and adverse-effect measures can be used for Team Breathe-Easy's work:

Process Measures

- COPD patients and their families who received education from a respiratory therapist on how to manage dyspnea at home.
- Staff members who could confidently describe the new discharge process for patients.
- Off-hours calls answered within 15 minutes.

Outcome Measures

- Rate of hospitalized COPD patients who are not readmitted within three months of hospital discharge.
- Rate of COPD patients on home oxygen who are not readmitted within three months of hospital discharge.

- Rates for ER use, as well as planned hospitalizations.
- Direct reports from patients about managing dyspnea at home.

Adverse-Effect Measures

- Frequency of on-call service not being able to get to the home within two hours (due to managing more and sicker patients at home).
- Frequency of patients leaving the practice because they are put off by requirements for self-management and ACP.

Team Breathe-Easy decided to collect outcome-measure data monthly and solicited reports of any adverse effects. They tracked the core outcome measure for one year.

Telling Your Story: Time Series Chart

Team Breathe-Easy

To measure progress, Team Breathe-Easy decided to chart how many hospitalized COPD patients were not *readmitted to the hospital or emergency room within three months of the patients' initial hospital discharge. This measure was appealing because it was so easy to gather. Some of the team wanted to survey patients, but they realized that serious dyspnea virtually always led to the emergency room. Thus, the burden of surveys seemed to add little insight. To measure improvement, Team Breathe-Easy compared its hospital's readmission rate to the readmission rate of all COPD patients in the multisite system. Data were charted monthly.*

For the numerator, Team Breathe-Easy used the number of patients who were not readmitted within three months of their initial discharge from the hospital. The denominator was the total number of patients that the team had enrolled.

The team tracked its results on the time series chart shown in Figure 5.1.

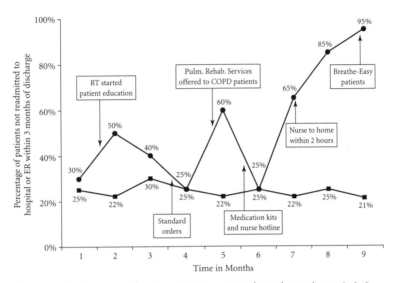

FIGURE 5.1 Team Breathe-Easy. ■–■–■, comparison site patients; ●–●–●, Breathe-Easy patients

IDENTIFYING AND TESTING CHANGES

TEAM BREATHE-EASY

The team began with three changes, which it introduced sequentially, over a three-month period. (Introducing all three changes at once would be too hard and would make it difficult to know which changes were worthwhile.) They eventually saw the need to try two more changes. The overall changes were the following:

1. *Having respiratory therapists educate patient and caregiver on specific self-care skills for the home.*

2. *Approving a new standard order sheet for drug treatment by the pulmonary physician.*
3. *Increasing referrals to pulmonary rehabilitation services.*
4. *Having medication kits at home and available by phone from the 24-hour nurse.*
5. *Arranging to have a nurse at the home within two hours of worsening symptoms.*

Team Breathe-Easy made each change on a small scale. For example, they trained one nurse to try out the new processes on a few patients and first worked out the standard order with one physician. By trying one change at a time, they gathered insight into which changes led to improvements. When they were satisfied that a change was working well and leading to improvement (after reviewing data), they spread the change to more patients, more doctors, and more units. In the first few months of the program, the team was disappointed to find that its readmission rates were not improving. Team members spent time on the unit, observing how the changes were being implemented, and talked with families at follow-up visits.

Here are some strategies for change that you can consider to improve symptom management in your organization.

- Consult specialists for particularly problematic situations, including the online advice available to clinicians through palliative care web boards such as http://growthhouse .net:8080/~growthhouse. (For access, you will need to create a user account or log-in as a guest.)
- Understand what the symptom means to the patient and the patient's family. (Is the symptom preventing other activities or disrupting family life?)

- Measure symptoms over time, and always follow up after changes in treatment.
- Incorporate symptom measurement in routine clinical management (e.g., pain as the "fifth vital sign").
- Use instruments designed for initial assessment of multiple symptoms (see the resources listed at the end of this chapter).
- Use focused instruments for monitoring specific symptoms.
- Use around-the-clock medication for continuous symptoms.
- Use medications appropriately, but also offer nonpharmaceutical treatments, including reassurance and refocusing.
- Be prepared to suppress almost any symptom with adequate opioids and sedatives if a patient who is near death would otherwise suffer greatly. Reassure the patient and family about this.

COMMON BARRIERS TO GOOD SYMPTOM MANAGEMENT

TEAM BREATHE-EASY

Initially, Team Breathe-Easy struggled to meet its goals. Within a few weeks, the group learned that self-care training would not yeild a re-admission rate of zero patients, no matter how rigorous or responsive the home management that was provided. Patients and families tended to panic when their efforts seemed to be failing and were unwilling to take chances by staying home. Instead, they continued to rush to the hospital. To counter this, the team developed a system to provide a 24-hour-nurse hotline and put medicine kits in the home to provide caregivers with resources to manage symptoms at home. While this improved things, families still felt anxious all the time and panicked after a few hours of trying to reverse deteriorating symptoms at home. This suggested the need to be able to promise to have a competent nurse at the home within two hours. Finally, ER visits decreased.

All improvement efforts encounter barriers. Anticipating and preparing for them will allow your team to overcome problems while simultaneously staying focused on your aim. Barriers associated with improving symptom management may include the following:

- Low expectations: accepting symptoms as inevitable.
- Inadequate knowledge: inadequate assessment and not being aware of treatment possibilities.
- Symptom measurement: some are hard to measure.
- Differing priorities of patient and family: sometimes, one worries about death and others about more suffering.
- Concern about side effects of medication.
- Reluctance to take opioid medications due to fear of addiction or sedation.

Most of these have a fairly obvious response, once you recognize that the problem exists. Set high goals, be sure you have expertise, educate everyone involved, and try things out on a small scale.

SOME SPECIAL CASES: OLDER OR COGNITIVELY IMPAIRED PATIENTS

According to the American Geriatrics Society Panel on Chronic Pain in Older Persons (1998, http://www.americangeriatrics.org/staging/education/executive_summ.shtml), chronic pain in the long-term care setting is generally underrecognized and undertreated. In addition, the ways in which older people communicate about their pain may be different. Older adults may deny that they are in pain if you ask them directly, "Are you in pain?" They may even appear to be comfortable, smiling and responsive, and still be very uncomfortable. Older adults may expect that they will have unpleasant symptoms in later life or be afraid of its consequences (more tests, another illness, more burdens on family). So it is important to use words that they may use to describe their pain, such as hurt, ache, discomfort, or sore: "Do you hurt anywhere?" may be a better way to ask about pain; and "What keeps you from enjoying the day?" may give insight into symptoms generally.

Older adults and others with cognitive impairments may still be able to respond to questions about their discomfort even with limited use of language skills. Ask yes-or-no questions, and ask the patient to point to what hurts.

When patients can not communicate about their symptoms, the healthcare practitioner has to find other ways to assess signs and symptoms of distress. You will have to depend on your other senses, your knowledge of how the person usually acts, and the insights of family and staff to determine whether a noncommunicative person is in distress.

Observe the patient for signs of rapid or distressed breathing, curled up body positioning, repetitive movements, or resistance to being moved or helped. The face may reveal grimacing, teeth clenching, tears, or eyes opened widely, all signals that the person is in distress.

Behaviors may change when the person is uncomfortable; the person may become loud, call out, be verbally or physically abusive, or be resistant to caregiving. Assess whether this has happened before and what might trigger this behavior (the need to urinate or move the bowels; being too cold or too hot; hunger; loneliness; fear of caregiving procedures; experiencing harmful stimuli from the environment). If the cause of the behavior is not identified, try pain-relief measures, and then observe to see whether the person acts and appears better after the treatment.

Some measurement tools allow aides to rate pain for people with dementia, including the PAIN AD Scale (see the resources listed at the end of this chapter).

GIVE THEM SOMETHING TO TALK ABOUT

TEAM BREATHE-EASY

Eventually, Team Breathe-Easy achieved its revised aim, and the project ended. However, the team wanted to be sure that staff did not revert to the old way of handling these very-ill patients. To maintain its gains, the team trained all current and new providers on the new protocols for symptom management by including the protocols in new employee orientation, in required in-service training, and in regular seminars. With the support of senior management, they made a new requirement for all respiratory therapists: RTs were required to make a follow-up phone call to each patient two days after discharge. They made extra efforts to update the home health nurse assigned to the patient on discharge. With everyone's help, the team sustained the changes and made them permanent.

Once Team Breathe-Easy had successfully implemented and sustained new symptom-management practices, they began sharing their success story with others throughout the organization, presenting their results in seminars and training sessions. Eventually, they published their story in a professional journal.

TOOLS AND RESOURCES

Symptom-Specific Treatment

A Starter Guide to Symptom-Specific Treatment

Symptom	Treatment Possibilities
Shortness of Breath Dyspnea	Change position.
	Use relaxation techniques.
	Improve airway circulation.
	Dispense medications: opioids, such as morphine;

A Starter Guide to Symptom-Specific Treatment (*continued*)

Symptom	Treatment Possibilities
	sedatives, such as benzodiazepines; oxygen; corticosteroids;or bronchodilators, as needed.
	Use a fan, which encourages the individual to feel that air is available.
	Unclutter the environment.
	Do not rush the patient, and allow for breaks for the patient to catch his or her breath during activities.
	Provide supplemental oxygen.
Fatigue	Conserve energy.
	Improve sleep.
	Exercise, or provide physical therapy.
	Dispense medications: psychostimulants; low-dose corticosteroids (e.g., dexamethasone or prednisone); antidepressants; trial of erythropoietin for fatigue caused by anemia.
	Provide rest periods between activities.
Dry Mouth	Drink lots of fluids, except in the active dying phase, when fluid intake might be detrimental.
	Maintain good oral hygiene.
	Provide humidified air.
	Suck on ice or vitamin C tablets.
	Chew sugarless gum.
	Use artificial saliva, provided in a spray form.
	Swab the mouth with cool water.
Appetite	Eat small, frequent meals.
	Eat high-calorie, high-protein foods, and take nutritional supplements.
	Obtain nutritional counseling.

A Starter Guide to Symptom-Specific Treatment (*continued*)

Symptom	Treatment Possibilities
	Trial of medication: corticosteroid, megestrol acetate, dronabinol, cyproheptadine, pentoxifylline.
Weight Loss	Protect the skin, provide for debility, try supplements, but accept weight loss as normal dying.
Nausea and Vomiting	Take antinausea medication.
	Snack on frequent light meals throughout the day.
	Avoid fried, spicy, or acidic foods.
	Maintain oral hygiene.
	Provide fresh air.
	Avoid strong odors.
	Provide rest and relaxation.
	Intake clear fluids.
Pressure Ulcers	Keep skin dry and clean.
	Check skin daily for pressure sores and other skin irritations.
	Turn a bedridden person every few hours, alternating positions.
	Keep the heels off the bed.
	Encourage the patient to get out of bed as much as possible.
	Never leave the patient lying or sitting in wet clothes or bedding.
	Make sure the bedding is not wrinkled or irritating the patient's skin.
	Promote a balanced, nutritious diet that is high in protein.
	Do not open or break blisters.

A Starter Guide to Symptom-Specific Treatment (*continued*)

Symptom	Treatment Possibilities
	Put dry, clean gauze on any open areas until a clinician can assess and provide appropriate dressings.
	Alternate pressure pad or special pressure-reducing mattress and seating pads.
Anxiety	Teach stress-management techniques, such as progressive relaxation, guided imagery, and hypnosis
	Provide counseling.
	Encourage support from family, friends, spiritual leaders, and peers.
	Maintain control of pain, side effects from medication and other medical conditions, where possible.
	Trial of medication: benzodiazepines, other tranquilizers (such as the phenothiazines and haloperidol), antihistamines (e.g., hydroxyzine), antidepressants, opioids.
Depression	Exercise, if able, including walking.
	Dispense antidepressant medication, including methylphenidate (when appropriate) for quick relief.
	Manage pain and other distressing symptoms.
	Provide counseling.
	Encourage support from spiritual leaders, family, friends, and peers found through support groups. Teach stress relief and pain management techniques, such as relaxation, guided imagery, and distraction.

Adapted from http://www.stoppain.org. Used with permission.

There are many instruments available for measurement of multiple symptoms (MSAS, Rotterdam Symptom Checklist, Symptom Distress Scale).

What Are the Best Symptom-Management Tools That I Can Use to Assess My Patients?

- Edmonton Symptom Assessment System (ESAS)
  http://www. palliative.org/PC/ClinicalInfo/AssessmentTools/
  esas.pdf
- Assessing Pain in People with Dementia
  http://www.hartfordign.org/publications/trythis/
  assessingPain.pdf
- Borg Scale (for assessment of dyspnea)
  http://www.promoting excellence.org/downloads/measures/
  borg_scale.pdf
- Memorial Symptom-Assessment Scale
  http://www.promotingexcellence.org/downloads/measures/
  memorial_symptom_assessment_scale.pdf

What Are Some Good Websites for Symptom-Management Resources?

- City of Hope
  http://mayday.coh.org
- Department of Pain and Palliative Care at Beth Israel Medical
  Center
  http://www.stoppain.org/
- Partners Against Pain
  http://www.partnersagainstpain.com/
- ICU Delirium and Cognitive Impairment Study Group
  http://www.icudelirium.org/delirium/
- Growth House
  http://www.growthhouse.org/

6

CARING FOR CAREGIVERS

IN THIS CHAPTER

- Caregivers' needs in serious illness and end-of-life care
- Interventions for advanced illness caregivers
- Setting goals that promote caregiver support
- Support for healthcare providers and staff

Family or volunteer caregivers make it possible to meet the needs of the long-term, medically complex patient. Approximately 25 million Americans provide care for a relative or friend who is unable to manage alone because of illness, disability, or frailty. Most of these family caregivers are middle-aged or older, and caregiving increases their risk for ill health and financial problems. Family members often assume the caregiving role under sudden and extreme circumstances, and caregivers frequently have little understanding about the patient's disease or how to provide care. Informal family caregiving involves a variety of direct care activities (i.e, activities carried out to assist the patient, such as bathing, eating, toileting, dressing, grooming, and emotional support) and indirect care (such as medication management, transportation, advocacy, supervision and management of paid care workers, coordination among healthcare providers, and assistance with medical bills and other finances). In addition, families provide complex care: they may manage symptoms, monitor clinical changes, administer medications, and operate high-technology equipment (i.e., infusion pumps or IVs).

While providing care for a disabled, frail, or seriously ill loved one can be rewarding, it also consumes time, money, and energy. Caregivers are at an increased risk for mental health problems, physical health problems, and death. To fulfill their demanding role, caregivers need information about disease progression, training in patient care, support for medical decision-making, financial help, respite care, and emotional and spiritual support. However, these needs have often been ignored (or misunderstood) by those in the healthcare system.

Although many factors influence how family caregivers respond to their role, managing advanced illness and the end of life is particularly stressful. Caregivers express fears of the future and often suffer depression and anxiety, deterioration of relationships, concern about the suffering of their loved one, and worries about how caregiving will affect their own health (e.g., fatigue, sleep deprivation, social life disruption, financial concerns, etc.). Our experience has shown that good quality improvement (QI) teams tailor their interventions to the needs of the caregivers and patients according to the care setting, the patient's disease stage, and the caregiver's situation. A few organizations have applied the QI model to support their caregivers. Some interventions reduce readmission rates while at the same time assisting caregivers. Others simply improve the caregivers' quality of life.

TEAM FAIRLAWN

A number of physicians and nurses on the Geriatric Management Team and one activist nurse from the intensive care unit (ICU) at Fairlawn Hospital met regularly to discuss patients under their inpatient and clinic care and to try to understand how well their system was delivering care for advanced illness and the end-of-life. In the busy rush of day-to-day patient management, the team did not feel that they had a good sense of the quality of care being provided across their hospital or across the system's many delivery sites. They had experienced problems in a variety of areas: the lack of completed advance care plans for seriously ill and dying patients; families being ignored or avoided if there were conflicts concerning goals of care between clinicians and family members; and little patient and caregiver support in the community for discharged patients. The team decided to do something about these problems. After some discussion, they decided to start in the hospital, where they had some control over the setting. They wanted to offer more holistic care for their patients and caregivers, including clinical caregivers. The question, then, was: What to do and where to start?

Identifying the Problem and Setting an Aim

You may have some sense of what the problems are for caregivers in your particular setting. Indeed, the needs are substantial. Providing supportive services to caregivers crosses almost all settings because so few organizations are doing much for caregivers. You may need to do some groundwork to get a better sense of what the most important problems are for your families. Obtaining baseline data from the caregivers of current and former patients may help you brainstorm. For example, follow-up phone calls to even a few (10–20) caregivers of patients recently discharged from your facility (e.g., high readmission CHF or COPD patients) will enable you to determine how the caregiver is managing in the community, what problems they are facing, and how the patient is doing after discharge. These calls may point out problems in discharge education and support; correcting these problems may result in improved patient care and lower readmissions. In addition, surveys of staff in particular settings (e.g., the ICU, the ER, dialysis clinics, etc.) regarding issues they see as problematic can illuminate areas for improvement. Once you have identified key issues, settle on at least one aim and decide how you will measure your improvement efforts.

TEAM FAIRLAWN

*Rather than acting on vague ideas, Team Fairlawn started survey-
ing clinicians in various hospital settings about their experience with
seriously ill and dying patients and how well clinicians felt they were
able to provide support and spend time with the family. In addition,
the QI team decided to make a few informal telephone calls to the
caregivers of recently deceased ICU/medical/surgery patients to learn
what might have been more helpful to the patient and family during
the last weeks and days. What they heard was not encouraging. While
family members stated that they felt the medical care at Fairlawn
was "good" for their loved one at the end, a majority of families reported the following.*

- *Their loved one was in pain or had severe shortness of breath at
  the end.*
- *They would have appreciated having alternative and complementary therapies available to their loved ones.*
- *They were not aware of the need for advance care planning
  (ACP), what the ACP discussions involved, and often felt left out
  of some decision-making or "talked down to" by clinicians.*
- *They were scared, did not know who was responsible for treating
  their loved one, and did not know what to do for their loved one.*
- *They did not have any time or place to be alone with their loved
  one and had to be on the hospital's schedule and not their loved
  one's.*
- *They were not given enough information, or in a timely enough
  manner, to make good decisions; they were guilt-ridden concerning treatment withdrawal decisions that they felt forced to
  make.*
- *They felt abandoned by clinical staff after the death of their loved
  one.*

- *They and/or the patient would have liked to have had spiritual or religious guidance offered or rituals performed.*
- *They were infuriated that the billing department continued to send medical bills to the family in the name of the deceased. They wanted to know whether anyone had told the billing department that the patient was dead.*

Team Fairlawn was impressed by what they learned from their baseline data collection and decided to fix as much of the problem over the course of nine months as they possibly could. They identified a series of interventions to achieve their broad goal of supporting caregivers. The next step was to set one overall aim statement that could help the team stay focused on their goals and help identify ways in which to measure progress. Team Fairlawn developed the following aim statement.

Aim: *Within nine months, Fairlawn Hospital will have implemented a Caregiver Support Services Program and provided services to 100% of targeted caregivers and to the clinical care team.*

What will improve: *Caregiver support services at Fairlawn Hospital.*
By how much: *One hundred percent served.*
By when: *Within nine months.*
For whom: *At-risk of death and dying patients, their families, and their clinicians.*

Some QI teams have assigned social workers or nurses to broker services within their healthcare system (e.g., enhanced geriatric care coordination programs) or created an Advanced Illness Doula Program, in which a trained volunteer or paid employee serves as a guide who links the families of dying patients with the facility's social, financial, and psychosocial/spiritual services. Other teams have provided a hospitality cart for families keeping vigil in the ICU, or a private room or kitchen facilities for families to use while their loved one is hospitalized. Some teams have worked to enhance the advance care planning, communication, and continuity skills of their clinical teams through role playing, educational materials, and monitoring. Still others have worked within the larger community to enhance awareness of end-of-life issues and develop community-wide strategies to improve caregiver support services, continuity, advance care planning, and end-of-life quality of care.

Barriers to Improved Caregiver Support

Virtually all improvement efforts encounter barriers. Anticipating and preparing for them will allow your team to overcome problems while staying focused on your aim. Institutional barriers that most teams face related to caregiver support include the following:

- Fear of getting involved in what may seem to be the limitless needs of families.
- Lack of familiarity with the everyday demands of caregiving.
- Lack of reliable resources to support caregivers.

Below is a list of the challenges that family caregivers often face.

- **Information and Communication:** A general lack of accurate, understandable, and timely information and communication between patients, families, and healthcare providers about the patient's illness and prognosis, treatment options, and what to expect next; a lack of availability of clinicians when families have questions; and poor communication among clinical providers within and across settings.
- **Advance Care Planning (ACP):** Dying patients often end up getting inappropriate and undesired aggressive treatment because there is no other plan; because completed plans are

not on record or no one is responsible for having them completed; because there is little standardization across settings as to what should be included in the ACP or ACP discussions; because facilities emphasize legal forms rather than more comprehensive care planning; and because providers are reluctant to bring up ACP because they do not feel confident that they will know what to say or how to respond (see Chapter 3, Advance Care Planning, for more details).

- **Continuity of Care:** There are often a lack of "common" or uniform plans of care across settings; a lack of communication among providers of vital elements of the care plan, including a list of problems, baseline physical, cognitive, and functional status, current medications and allergies, and caregiver contact information; a lack of preparation for the goals of care in the next setting; a lack of explicit arrangements for follow-up appointments, laboratory testing, and reconciliation of medication regimens; a lack of timely and appropriate follow-up from one setting to another to ensure that the care plan is properly and fully executed; a lack of preparation of the patient and caregiver for transitions, including problems with the transportation of the patient; and a lack of formal training in continuity/transitional care as a core competency for clinicians caring for elders who are frail and have advanced illness (see Chapter 7, "Continuity and Transfers," for more details).

- **Emotional, Psychosocial, Spiritual Support:** Clinicians often fail to refer caregivers to individual and group counseling and support services that include other caregivers in similar situations to address the emotional and psychological issues of caregivers.

- **Education/Training for Patient Management:** There may also be a lack of individualized and multicomponent education, information, and training and follow-up programs to enhance problem-solving/coping skills, meet patient medical needs, and assist the caregiver in patient behavior management (see Chapter 5 on CHF/COPD care and Chapter 10 on dementia care for more details of patient and caregiver support in the community).

- **Access to Support Services:** Clinicians may not refer caregivers to community resources for caregiver support services, such as respite services, financial counseling or assistance, and other social and health services needed by the family.

- **End-of-Life Care/Palliative Care/Supportive Care:** Caregivers often do not know about palliative or comfort care support services for the patient and supportive care services for the caregiver during the end of the loved one's life.

- **Follow-Up Bereavement Support:** Caregivers often do not have follow-up, bereavement referral/counseling, and psychosocial/spiritual support (see Chapter 14 on bereavement support for more details).

Choosing a Team

Team Fairlawn

Team Fairlawn decided to start by improving the team meetings and family conferences for patients and caregivers. The team would need to involve participants from the medical/surgery ward. In addition, if they wanted to designate a space for family meetings or for use by the families, they needed administrative leadership. If they were going to enhance access to clinicians for family caregivers, they needed a few physicians or nurse practitioners from the ward to get involved in the project. They realized that some projects might require assistance from the hospital's education, public relations, and information technology (IT) departments. The team began assigning the responsibility for recruitment of new team members and responsibility for the development and testing of each sequential step of the "Caregiver Support Services Program."

For your project to succeed, your team must include key players who can help you reach your aims. Depending on what your issues are, you should try to include people involved in the current flow of care processes. Try to limit your core team to six to eight people, but if you have a complex aim or an aim that has many components, establish subteams to focus on different parts of the project (see Chapter 2 for more details on team formation).

Caregiver education, continuity, psychosocial, and support services should be provided in all care settings. Each of the suggested interventions can be applied in a hospital or a nursing home, and some of them can also be applied in home health care. It is up to your team to determine what elements of a valuable caregiver support program are relevant for your setting now and what you can work toward for the future. Think about the key players in your system or in the community, and consider how they might work with your team.

Measuring Your Success

Tracking progress is key to understanding the effects of your efforts. It is also important when you need to tell your story to administrators and colleagues, often to gain their support. Whatever your aim, three basic measures (see Chapter 2, Basics of Quality Improvement, for more details) are the kinds of things you will count to determine the following.

- Whether you are implementing your changes systematically and appropriately (system process measures).
- Whether you are improving care (patient and family outcome measures).
- Whether your changes are causing unintended or negative consequences (adverse-effect measures).

Your team needs to decide which data to collect, who will be responsible for collecting it, and how often to collect it. Depending on how big your patient population is, you might want to establish a sampling plan to get unbiased, yet manageable, data. You also need to figure out how to display your data: daily, weekly, every two weeks, monthly, or quarterly. Weekly measurement is best, as it provides quick turnaround of information to track progress, but be sure you have enough patients to do so (usually, five patients per week are enough to measure weekly). If you have too few patients to measure weekly, then try every other week. Only measure those things on a quarterly basis that are long-term outcome measures or that can only be collected quarterly. In addition, be sure to collect enough data to build your case (or to see quickly when an improvement is not working).

Team Fairlawn

The team identified the following sub-aim.

Sub-aim: *Within six months, 100% of families/caregivers of patients who are at-risk of dying in our medical/surgery ward will have participated in an enhanced family conference/team meeting, within 72 hours of admission, with the multidisciplinary clinical care team.*

Consequently, Team Fairlawn decided to track the following measures.

Process measure: *Percent of target patient families for whom the enhanced multidisciplinary team/family meeting was conducted within 72 hours of admission to the ward.*

Outcome measure: *Percent of the target patient families participating in the enhanced multidisciplinary team/family meeting who express satisfaction because the team did the following:*

- *Provided clear, comprehensive information on the patient's current clinical status, prognosis, potential treatment choices (including palliative care), and survival issues.*

- *Discussed the possible use of time-limited trials for aggressive treatments and the criteria to establish when to stop them.*

- *Had a discussion with the patient and/or family resulting in a plan of care, with treatment goals; advance care plans for all likely contingencies; and a time frame for treatment trials.*

- *Offered the family Caregiver Support Services (including basic logistics information, access to social services and clergy, volunteer support, 24/7 access to the patient, and the "Caregiver Comfort Care Cart"), and provided written materials on these services for future reference.*

- *Gave the family a packet with information on facility protocols, local resources, referral services, local lodging, restaurants, and volunteers.*

- *Identified a single person on whom the family could rely for continuity of information.*

- *Ensured that clinicians spoke to families and caregivers respectfully, in clear language, that they provided sufficient time for the meeting, and that they listened to each family's concerns and values and made each family feel part of the team.*

- *Made certain that families found these meetings helpful or very helpful in understanding their loved one's medical situation, treatment options, and what they might expect next.*

Adverse-effect measure: *Percent of the target patients' families participating in the enhanced multidisciplinary team/family meeting who expressed greater confusion, anxiety, depression, or other negative feelings because of the meeting and/or who expressed that many of their questions remained unanswered and unsettled.*

To address other components of the project, a few team members also focused on reviewing and collecting baseline data on how family meetings were currently conducted by staff on the medical/surgery ward. They sampled five team meetings over the course of a week to observe the interaction and take notes on the content of information provided to families. They then asked families to describe what they had learned in the meetings and what questions they had. Another group of team members reviewed all printed materials that the medical/surgery ward currently gave to family members about local resources. (Many patients and caregivers came from surrounding areas and were unfamiliar with the city.) A third group collected baseline data on 15 recently deceased patients in the medical/surgery ward and studied what kind of advance care planning had been documented in each patient's record and whether the patient's and family's wishes were honored. They spoke to 10 caregivers of deceased patients to ask them about the experience and how the facility might have helped them more. They agreed to meet again in one week with results from their baseline data collection to review the information and identify next steps.

Following are some other examples of measures of caregiver support measures:

Process Measures

- Family members who participate in an enhanced clinical team/family conference meeting within 72 hours of the patient's admission.

- Clinical team/family conference meetings in which standard-ized guidelines, protocols, forms, and scripts for clinicians developed to enhance the meetings were used.
- The number of times that caregivers called the 24/7 access number for information or advice in a crisis and who received a prompt response (e.g., within one hour).
- Caregivers' needs assessed using a brief, standardized tool.
- Caregivers with identified needs promptly referred to an appropriate service provider or providers (e.g., for counseling, support groups, clergy, financial assistance, etc.) and followed up within 48 hours of referral.
- Caregivers able to identify the clinical team contact provider.
- Caregivers who received a follow-up bereavement contact within three months of a loved one's death and who were assessed for bereavement adjustment.
- Staff participating in facility-sponsored grief/bereavement support services.
- Caregivers provided with palliative and supportive care.

Outcome Measures

- Caregivers participating in the enhanced clinical team meetings or family conferences who were satisfied with the process using program-specific satisfaction measures.
- Caregivers who found family conferences helpful or very helpful in understanding their loved one's medical situation, treatment options, and what they should expect.
- Caregivers provided with respite care or psychosocial/ spiritual support services who state that such services were very helpful.
- Caregivers using the "comfort care cart" or "family room/ kitchen" who stated that these services were very helpful during their loved one's illness.

- Caregivers who say that they knew what to expect and had no surprises during the patient's final illness.
- Caregivers receiving education and training for patient management in the home who say they felt confident that they knew what to do, what to expect, and whom to contact with questions.
- Caregivers and staff attending a facility-based memorial service for recently deceased patients who state that the program was helpful to them.
- Caregivers referred to and followed up with by facility clergy for spiritual support.
- Caregivers provided with palliative/support care who state that the services were helpful.

Adverse-Effect Measures

- Caregivers who find the clinical team meeting or family conference troublesome or painful.
- Staff who stated that providing enhanced caregiver support services added a significant burden to their workday.
- Staff who stated that using QI strategies to improve clinical care added a significant burden to their workday.
- Patients who are hospitalized or placed in the facility who do not receive ACP discussions within 72 hours of admission.
- Staff who stated that they felt unprepared to handle the family conference due to inadequate preparation or training.
- Caregivers who felt unprepared for a transition to the home or for how to manage once their loved one was home.
- Caregivers who stated that managing care for their loved one after discharge increased their anxiety, depression, or burden.

TELLING YOUR STORY: TIME SERIES GRAPH

TEAM FAIRLAWN

*To measure progress, Team Fairlawn charted at least one process mea-
sure: how many of its target patient caregivers participated in their
enhanced clinical team/family conference meetings within 72 hours of
admission (see Figure 6.1). Team Fairlawn tracked caregiver satisfaction with the enhanced services support, an outcome measure (see Figure 6.2).*

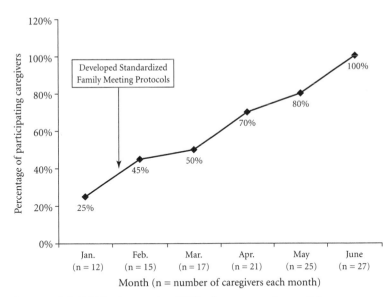

FIGURE 6.1 Within six months, 100% of target caregivers will have
participated in a family conference within 72 hours of admission.

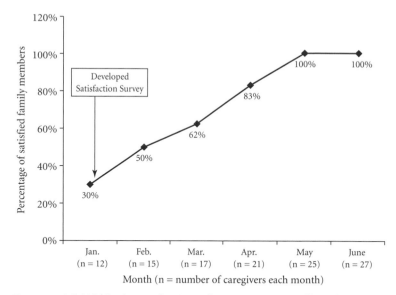

FIGURE 6.2 Within six months, 80% of target caregivers will say that they found family meetings "useful" or "very helpful."

IDENTIFYING AND TESTING CHANGES

Caregivers have vastly different needs at various points in a loved one's illness. No single intervention seems to address every need. To fill this gap, many programs now take a comprehensive, multifaceted approach to caregiver support by offering a range of community services and specific caregiving interventions. Programs have included elements such as four-hour weekly respite care, weekly caregiver-focused health-care visits, education on self-care after a death, and monthly support group meetings. There are many opportunities in today's healthcare environment to assist and support caregivers, whether in the community after hospital discharge, in rehabilitation or nursing facilities, or in the hospital (see Chapter 7 on continuity of care/transfers, and see Chapter 10 on dementia).

INTERDISCIPLINARY CARE TEAMS

Advanced illness patients benefit most from multidisciplinary care: they do better when all team members (professionals, paraprofessionals, and volunteers) feel that they are equally valued, can offer ideas and recommendations, and be heard. Team members must communicate, review their work together, work out problems and barriers, and share successes and failures. A team-building focus can pay off in increased effectiveness and productivity (through less confusion about assignments, fewer misunderstandings, and shared responsibility), greater patient and/or staff satisfaction and quality of care, and fewer conflicts among staff. Team-building strategies include the following:

- Write a mission and purpose statement with participation and goal setting by the team.
- Establish defined roles and responsibilities for team members.
- Develop conflict-management procedures.
- Improve the team's communication and problem-solving skills/strategies.
- Develop respect, if not actual friendship, among team members.
- Conduct effective interdisciplinary team meetings reviewing patient care (e.g., discuss experiences with patients and families, review patient status and problems, address conflict resolution).
- Build morale through staff-directed teams and staff decision-making, open communication, open-door management, cohesion among staff, and high levels of autonomy and self-direction.
- Provide support through recognition and celebration of individuals and teams and their accomplishments; create opportunities for staffers to share their experiences.

- Provide bereavement, counseling, and grief support for staff through psychosocial support services, as well as institution-supported memorial services for deceased patients for staff and families.

Employee Advancement and Continuing Education

All professionals are interested in advancing their careers, but the path may not be clear. Nursing shortages and high turnover rates for paraprofessional staff require strategies to help employees find satisfaction with their current positions while pursuing opportunities for advancement. One useful way to do this is to offer employees ongoing training and education programs. Some organizations have improved retention of nurses and certified nursing assistants by offering classes and programs to enhance professional caregiving skills. With support and encouragement, paraprofessionals often can also advance in nursing or allied health professions, such as administration, grief counseling, emergency medical services, and chaplaincy.

Clinician and Staff Support

Healthcare providers are also caregivers, and they face numerous stresses in helping patients, families, and other clinicians address the important medical, social, spiritual, and emotional issues of serious illness and the end of life. Staff must routinely provide an intense level of care. Current realities, such as having to see more patients in less time, make developing long-term, trusting relationships with patients and their families especially challenging. The challenge can lead to provider burnout. Staff need recognition and acknowledgment of the hard work of the complex patient care that they offer. Moreover, the death of a patient affects paid as well as family and volunteer caregivers.

Many clinicians and staff may need time and rituals to acknowledge a patient's death and to pay tribute to the patient and family. Some QI teams have focused on reducing staff burden and found that it leads to improved morale and staff retention. Clinical and support staff areas ripe for improvement include the following.

- Building interdisciplinary care teams.
- Employee advancement and continuing education.
- Institution-supported counseling, support groups, and memorial services for staff.

Give Them Something to Talk About

Practical Changes to Support Caregivers

- Multidisciplinary team management of advanced illness and "at-risk of death" patients in the hospital, nursing home, and community setting, including social work, clergy, and volunteers to enhance continuity and support.
- Caregiver assessment and follow-up regarding support needs (e.g., spirituality, counseling, bereavement/grief support).
- Timely and comprehensive family meetings, to be conducted with the entire multidisciplinary care team and family within 48 hours of admission, to discuss patient status, treatment goals, and advance care plans.
- Twenty-four-hour, seven-days-per-week telephone access to one consistent member of the care team for families to contact when they have questions, need to talk, or want to check in with the healthcare team.
- Comprehensive caregiver education, skills, and coping training; provision of information materials; and in-person follow-up for all advanced illness patients discharged into

the community within 72 hours of discharge. Training programs include didactic instruction, role-play, corrective feedback, and data collection designed to improve caregiver skills.

- A private room or space on each floor that families can use when visiting their loved ones.
- A comfort care/palliative care hospitality cart for patients and families.
- Individual counseling or support group interventions for caregivers and staff.
- Respite care with services available to caregivers for some periods of relief from caregiving, including daily attendance at adult daycare; short-term, in-home companion services; volunteer assistance; and hospice care.
- Availability of complementary and alternative therapies for patients and families, such as massage therapy, therapeutic touch, music therapy, aromatherapy, and yoga.
- A patient diary by the patient's bedside so that staff may write notes or messages about the patient that the family can keep when the patient dies.
- Stamped envelopes and bereavement cards and notepaper kept at the nurses' station for clinicians and staff to sign or to write a letter to the deceased patient's family after the death.
- Regular memorial services and counseling and support opportunities held for families, caregivers, and clinicians and staff.
- A volunteer-run "Angel by the Bedside" program to provide a companion, so that no patient dies alone.
- Systematic personal follow-up of family members of recently deceased patients for satisfaction, problem assessment, referral, and counseling or support group services.

Tools and Resources

- National Family Caregiver Support Program (NFCSP),
  Administration on Aging (AoA), U.S. Department of Health
  and Human Services (HHS)
  http://www.aoa.dhhs.gov/prof/aoaprog/caregiver/overview/
     overview_caregiver.asp
- Family Caregiver Alliance
  http://www.caregiver.org
- Aging Parents and Elder Care
  http://www.aging-parents-and-elder-care.com
- American Association of Retired Persons
  http://www.aarp.org
- Caregiver Support (a gateway to a number of other caregiver
  resources)
  http://www.vitalco.net/Caregiver.htm
- National Alliance for Caregiving
  http://www.caregiving.org
- Caring Connections
  http://www.caringinfo.org

7

CONTINUITY AND TRANSFERS

IN THIS CHAPTER

- Issues in transitions of care (across settings and among providers)
- Barriers to continuity of care
- Important components of continuity of care
- Changes that improve continuity of care:
  - transitions between different levels of care in the same facility
  - transitions between hospital and community or home settings
  - transitions between nursing facilities and hospitals

Advanced illness near the end of life makes patients especially vulnerable to errors during transitions from one setting or provider to another. These shortcomings in healthcare compound problems for patients and organizations. Poorly implemented transitions account for a significant portion of medical errors, service duplication, and unnecessary utilization. Many transitions are unplanned or unanticipated. Many occur on nights and weekends when the regular clinicians may not be easily accessible. Essential information about the patient's problems and care plan is often lost between care settings. Families and patients may be confused by conflicting recommendations from different healthcare providers; they may encounter multiple payment systems and unfamiliar providers across settings. The complex medication and monitoring regimens associated with most chronic illnesses carry a high potential for error, missed treatments, and duplication. Transitions cause tremendous adjustment problems for older adults who may be frail, cognitively impaired, or alone. Patients may also suffer from a lack of follow-up care, and they and their caregivers are frequently unprepared for what to expect in the new care setting. The benefit of transferring a patient must be weighed against such costs.

Continuity of care is more than discharge planning or utilization management. It is defined as a set of actions that ensure the coordination and continuity of healthcare as patients transfer between different locations or different levels of care within the same location (e.g., hospital ward to rehabilitation). Continuity is the degree to which a series of discrete healthcare events is experienced as coherent and connected with the patient's medical and human needs; it is distinguished by two core elements: care over time and care for the individual.

In this chapter, we present tips on how to apply quality improvement (QI) in your setting to promote better care across settings. The story of Team Oakwood, a composite of teams which have successfully used QI methods to improve continuity of care and transitions, will help guide you through this process.

TEAM OAKWOOD

Problems in transitions between hospitals, the community, and their local nursing facilities hit home for staff at Oakwood Hospital when the mother of Oakwood's director of nursing (DON) was discharged home after an acute episode. The patient had advanced heart failure and was slightly demented; her husband, although intellectually sound, was growing frail and could not manage his wife at home on his own.

The director was out of town when her mother came to the emergency room. Although the DON knew her own system well, she found it hard to coordinate her mother's care, even in the hospital. Important clinical information was missing from her mother's medical record, and her advance care plan had been left at home. Although the hospital care itself was fine, her parents received little planning, follow-up, or support after their discharge. No one called to follow-up during her mother's first few days home. Her mother became confused about medications and had difficulty moving around her home. Her father's frailty made it difficult for him to help his wife. Her mother missed a follow-up appointment with her primary-care physician because it was not included in her discharge instructions. When she did see her doctor, he was unaware that she had been hospitalized. Her physician discovered that she had been prescribed new medications that were contraindicated and could have caused complications. In the past, the DON had heard complaints from the ER staff about missing information on patients being transferred to the hospital from Oakwood's partner nursing facility. This missing information resulted in errors or in extra time needed to obtain current medication lists and advance care plans from the nursing home. The DON decided these transitions and continuity-of-care issues were problems she wanted to take on for Oakwood Hospital.

IDENTIFYING THE PROBLEM AND SETTING AN AIM

You may know what the problem is in your particular setting—medical records that are not transferred quickly enough to another setting, advance care plans that are not in the chart, or the transfer of dying patients—but not know precisely how to solve it. Or you may need to do some groundwork to gather information before pinpointing a problem that is suited to a rapid-cycle change process. In either case, you do not want to spend so much time gathering data or getting input that you ultimately do nothing. Instead, collect baseline data—just enough to see where the problem is but not enough to publish a research paper. In the hospital setting, you might start by focusing on the following:

- "Frequent fliers" (patients who return to the hospital soon after discharge).
- Large diagnostic groups, such as patients with advanced heart failure or chronic obstructive pulmonary disease.
- Nursing home residents who arrive in your ER or admissions office without advance care plans.
- Reliability of handoffs among different levels of care within your setting.

Some teams find that small discussion groups of five or six people (staff, patients, family members) are an effective way to learn more about what is happening.

TEAM OAKWOOD

The director of nursing gathered a few unit nurses and other colleagues. The team spent a month talking to stakeholders: discharge planning social workers, ER nurses, the medical director of the closest nursing home, and a few recently discharged patients and their caregivers. The team analyzed readmission data to identify the problems that may have caused the readmissions. Based on these activities, the team decided to start with "frequent fliers" and to work toward the involvement of their local home health agencies and nursing facilities. The team settled on a few changes to test. They started with uniform medication lists and discharge forms that patients could take to all subsequent healthcare providers. Next, the team developed a care management/transition coach intervention and continuity-of-care guidelines and protocols. In addition, the team wanted to improve transfers between local nursing facilities and Oakwood's ER by developing standardized transition care plans that included all the needed information for smooth transitions and continuity of care. The team recruited a number of Oakwood staff, as well as several stakeholders and providers from outside the hospital. These discussions led them to develop the following aim.

Aim: *Within nine months, 100% of transferred frail or demented patients' family caregivers or the post-discharge setting health care providers will report that Oakwood Hospital provided full and accurate transfer information that resulted in a safe, error-free transfer.*

What will improve: Information transfer and safe, error-free transitions. By when: Within nine months. By how much: One hundred percent. For whom: Discharged frail elders or demented patients.

With your team, you need to specify one or more aims and get to work on the one that is most important or most likely to yield improvement (see Chapter 2 for a full discussion of the components of a good aim statement).

COMMON BARRIERS TO CONTINUITY OF CARE

As you work to improve continuity of care for your patients, you will encounter barriers. Do not be disheartened; instead, expect barriers and be prepared to overcome them. Following is a list that presents common obstacles to continuity of care.

Barriers in Current Site of Care

- No plan of care, transition checklist, or medication lists across settings.
- No summary of the care provided by the sending institution.

- No communication of vital elements of the care plan among providers.
- No preparation for the goals of care in the next setting.
- No reconciliation of the patient's previous medications with the current regimen.
- No explicit arrangements for follow-up appointments.
- No reporting of laboratory testing.
- No timely and appropriate follow-up from one setting to another to ensure that the care plan is properly and fully executed.
- No preparation of the patient and family for transitions, including:
  a. patient and family support;
  b. education for symptom and disease management;
  c. information about what to expect in the next care setting.
- No explicit training of patients and families about how to respond to the patient's changing needs.

Barriers Between Sites of Care

- No education or support in the community for the patient's self-management and the family's management of a chronic condition.
- No shared information systems across sites.
- No ready availability of the patient's advance care plan for all healthcare sites.
- No formal training in continuity/transitional care for frail elders and advanced illness patients.

Choosing a Team

You have already identified a problem, created at least one aim statement, and identified a patient population for which to start testing changes. For your project to succeed, your team must include key players. Depending on your program's issues, you should try to include important people who are involved in the current flow of the care processes. Try to limit the team to six to eight people; but if you have a complex aim or one with many components, include subteams to focus on different aspects of the project. For example, recruit a clinician who is close to the patients in your target population. Include an organizational leader, someone skilled in QI, and someone willing to do the day-to-day work (see Chapter 2 for more details on team building).

TEAM OAKWOOD

The team decided to focus on its frail and demented patients first. To do this, they needed one or two friendly clinicians on a ward to participate in the project. They also needed to involve clerks and volunteers to help gather baseline information. Eventually, they wanted to provide true continuity across settings, so the team worked to involve home health providers, hospital discharge planners, and care coordinators.

MEASURING SUCCESS

Tracking progress helps you to understand the effects of your efforts and to tell your story to administrators, colleagues, and funders. Measures help to determine:

- whether you are implementing the changes you want to make systematically and appropriately (process measures);
- whether you are improving care (outcome measures); and
- whether changes are causing unintended consequences or negative consequences (adverse-effect measures).

TEAM OAKWOOD

The team tracked the following measures.

Process measure: *Percent of discharged frail or demented patients with completed continuity-of-care information sheets transferred with them at discharge (as measured by the hospital discharge provider in a follow-up survey).*

Outcome measure: *Percent of discharged frail or demented patients who had an error-free transfer, as measured by a follow-up physician or caregiver.*

Adverse-effect measure: *Percent of discharged frail or demented patients' caregivers who state that they were unprepared for the transfer home or had problems after the discharge, as measured by a follow-up survey.*

Team Oakwood developed a plan to survey patients or caregivers, along with the staff at the facilities. The team defined frailty as hospitalized patients 80 years or older or patients who had a diagnosis of dementia. They then identified the hospital ward clerks as the team members who could help to collect data to monitor progress (process measures) and how well the project was working for patients and providers (outcome and adverse-effect measures).

The team identified data collection procedures. The hospital ward clerks would conduct a telephone survey of discharge planners within six hours after discharge to determine if the continuity-of-care information sheet was completed and forwarded to the patient or caregiver. One to three days after discharge, clerks would call the discharged patient's family caregiver or appropriate receiving facility provider (e.g., nursing home admissions clerk and/or providers) to determine whether the continuity-of-care information sheet had arrived with the patient and whether the transfer was error free. The clerks received a free lunch for every pair of completed surveys. Completed surveys were sent electronically to the QI department, which analyzed data on a weekly basis, recording the number of eligible discharged patients; the next care setting; the number of pairs of on-site and follow-up surveys completed; and the number of patients discharged home with no problems noted. The team monitored completion rates but graphed on their run chart the rate of "no problem/error-free transfers" among discharges. The survey also monitored reports of problems. After reviewing the first test cycle data, Team Oakwood tweaked their processes to accommodate what did and did not work well in the first cycle test. They began to include a contact e-mail address and phone number on the continuity-of-care information sheet, asking caregivers to provide comments to the team on the continuity of care through the transfer. They then plotted results on time series graphs.

Irrespective of care setting, your measures must have a numerator (e.g., number of patients who completed the intervention) and a denominator (total number of patients for which the transition intervention was appropriate; Chapter 2 includes more details about measurement). The following lists present some examples of improved continuity-of-care and transition measures.

Process Measures

- Family caregivers who participate in an "enhanced" clinical team meeting or family conference within 72 hours of admission (or within 48 hours, if an ICU admission).
- Transferred target patients/residents with a completed, uniform transition form or care plan at discharge.
- Discharged target patients and caregivers who completed a standardized discharge education session 24 hours prior to hospital discharge.

- Patients and/or caregivers who maintain and update the personal health record (e.g., the Red Folder) over successive healthcare encounters.
- Family caregivers assessed for psychosocial/spiritual needs.
- Family caregivers referred to facility- or community-based services based on the caregiver assessment.

Outcome Measures

- Patients readmitted within seven days of initial discharge or transfer because of a transfer problem.
- Patients and families who state that they felt prepared to manage the transition thanks to education and support from the healthcare team.
- Patients' new providers who state that they had sufficient information about the patient and what had happened in prior care settings because of effective information transfer and communication with the previous team.
- Patients whose transitions are error free.
- Reduction in ER, ward, or nursing home processing time of transferred patients or residents due to standardized transfer forms and procedures across settings (e.g., time from admission to treatment using transfer information; reduction in follow-up calls for information; etc.).

Adverse-Effect Measures

- Patients, residents, and/or families who state that what happened during and after a transition was not what they were led to expect.
- Patients, residents, and/or caregivers who felt overwhelmed by the information and training.
- Documents accompanying transferred patients which include significant errors in treatment information.

TELLING YOUR STORY: TIME SERIES GRAPHS

TEAM OAKWOOD

The team prioritized its aims and began by working with patients and caregivers to help them become their own healthcare advocates. At-risk patients about to be discharged from the team leader's unit were identified and encouraged to participate. The team developed a draft transfer sheet that the patient and caregiver could take with them in a "Red Folder." Initial QI cycles showed the first form to be too cumbersome to complete prior to transfer; it was unclear whose responsibility it was to complete it. The team regrouped and looked at its early data and then worked with local primary-care providers to refine the transfer form so as to ensure that relevant information was being included for their use. Eventually, a standardized set of easily completed forms was tested and found to work. Patients and caregivers actually took the folder to subsequent healthcare visits, and the information was useful to other providers in planning care for these patients. Patients, caregivers, and providers found the Red Folder project very helpful. Figure 7.1 presents one of the time series charts that Team Oakwood developed for its administrators.

The team tracked whether the provider in the next healthcare setting saw the target patient's Red Folder and then used information in it for subsequent care recommendations. Figure 7.2 presents the outcome-data time series chart for this measure.

IDENTIFYING AND TESTING CHANGES

Three elements contribute to providing the right care in the right place at the right time:

1. providing accurate and current information about the patient across settings;

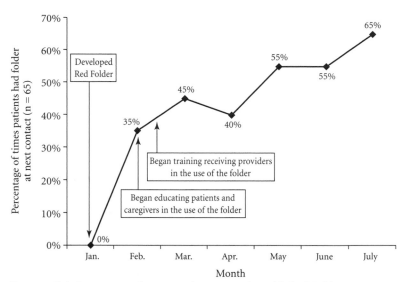

FIGURE 7.1 Percentage of target patients returning with Red Folder to next healthare visit

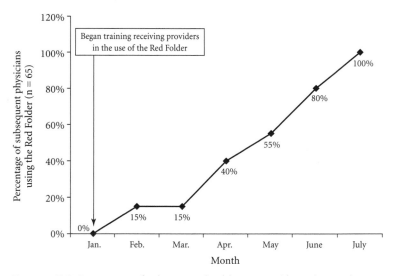

FIGURE 7.2 Percentage of subsequent healthcare providers who used information in Red Folder to establish patients' health care plans (n = 65)

2. having healthcare practitioners who understand complex, acute, and chronic care management and prioritize continuity of care;
3. enabling continuity of relationships among settings, patients, and families so as to bridge past and future care.

The following lists provide examples of changes tried by other teams. Use their specific suggestions to generate ideas on continuity-of-care improvements that you can make in your setting.

Continuity of Information

Regional use of standardized transfer forms, checklists, and/or care plans and uniform transfer protocols to ensure complete, accurate information transfer across care settings, including:

- A description of acute medical problems, including vital signs and exam, and a summary of all care provided to date, including procedures performed and their results.
- Functional baseline information.
- A list of current medications administered, including allergies.
- A complete summary of nursing home/hospital course (e.g., last 72 hours' graphics/vital signs), recent progress notes, and lab data.
- Any new treatments, including dressing changes, catheters, oxygen, diet/tube feedings.
- Five days of pre-transfer physician orders.
- All ACPs/directives transferred with the patient.
- Upcoming follow-up appointments with list of physicians' and caregivers' contact information.

Preparation for the patient, caregiver, and staff about what to expect includes the following:

- Education, counseling, and training sessions that teach the patient and/or caregiver about warning signs and symptoms that indicate a worsening condition.

- Direct communication and systematic information sharing among staff, including across different care settings.
- Regular review of any errors, near misses, or opportunities for improvement.
- Addition of a Transition Coach/Care Coordinator or *doula* to manage patient transitions and follow-ups.

Continuity of Care Management

An interdisciplinary geriatrics team that manages care, assigned to all frail, chronically ill, or nursing facility residents transferred to the hospital or admitted to the ER using standardized protocols for care management and communication. The facility focuses on:

- Maintaining the patient's cognitive and functional status.
- Treating the medical problem.
- Preventing pressure ulcers, constipation or fecal impaction, or the development of delirium.
- Avoiding Foley catheters (or removing them as soon as possible).
- Avoiding restraints.
- Attending to patients' oral fluid intake and nutrition.
- Offering frequent assisted walking or physical therapy to preserve mobility.

The care team focuses on the following:

- Providing timely, accurate, and sensitive communication of information with family and staff at all facilities involved in a patient's care.
- Standardizing care processes that anticipate and address patient and family needs *prior* to transitions.
- Assessing caregivers and assisting with care planning.
- Providing respite care: creating a family room or kitchen for

families whose loved ones have long-term needs; offering referrals for physical, psychosocial, and spiritual needs.

Continuity of Provider Relationships

Improved continuity and coordination of care for residents upon return to a nursing facility or home care through improved communication enabled by the following:

- Continuity of care provided by the same clinicians across settings to bridge past-to-current care and link to future care (e.g., the team follows the patient across settings).
- Development of a standardized transfer database to include all of the above information.
- Regular review of any errors, near misses, or opportunities for improvement.
- Regular meetings for staff at all facilities to collaborate, review processes, and identify and review transition or continuity errors.
- Regional, IT-based transfer information system for shared provider access.

GIVE THEM SOMETHING TO TALK ABOUT

Patients and caregivers have the power to help you improve continuity and transfers. While very sick people and their loved ones are not always in a position to advocate for their own needs, they can take control of essential healthcare information, becoming their own healthcare advocate and thus a partner in their healthcare team. By involving the patient and caregiver in managing their own care, clinicians can increase patient/caregiver knowledge and confidence and can reduce errors. Some QI teams have given their target patients copies of their current medical documents in a special folder (such as the Red Folder) to be updated in each care setting. Making the patient/caregiver responsible for the information and for its continual updating can improve their care. Patients learn to take the folder with them to any healthcare visit. Giving the patient or family this responsibility helps to enhance continuity of care. Some of our teams have had 90% of patients/caregivers bring the folder to the next healthcare visit and have had positive feedback from patients, caregivers, and providers about the use of the folders.

RED FOLDER: INFORMATION FOR PATIENTS TO TAKE TO FUTURE HEALTHCARE VISITS

- Health history, advance directives, physicians' contact information.
- Current medication list and allergies.
- Updated problem list and summary of care provided in the previous setting.
- Uniform care plan with current treatment goals and priorities, symptom-control measures, supportive services, and advance care plans.
- Baseline functional and cognitive testing and needs for assistance.
- Psychosocial and spiritual priorities.
- Documented information for the patient and caregiver on warning signs and symptoms and contact phone number.
- Caregiver assessment, environmental assessment, and current caregiver and provider contact information.

Other teams provided caregivers with stickers listing one contact person's telephone number. Some have instituted postdischarge follow-up using a transition coach/care coordinator for the first 72 hours after hospital discharge to reinforce hospital-based training in medication management, provide home situation assessment, and gauge how well patients and caregivers are coping.

We have found that groups working to improve transfers from hospital to home can focus on a few high-leverage strategies. The following list expands on some well-tested strategies for improving continuity across any setting.

1. Avoid transitions of very sick, old, or frail persons whenever possible.

2. Offer transition education, skills training, and follow-up support before discharge/transfer. This might include a series of face-to-face visits and telephone calls with a trained volunteer or nurse in the hospital prior to discharge and at home after discharge that is designed to teach self-management, to know red-flag signs and symptoms, and to understand medication schedules.

3. Give patient a portable personal health record (e.g., Red Folder) for use in future healthcare encounters. Include accurate, up-to-date, and comprehensive clinical, functional, and medication information that the patient can take from one provider to another.

4. Add a transition coach to the facility-based multidisciplinary healthcare provider team. For example, an advanced practice nurse intensively integrates and coordinates care with community-based providers during the transition between hospital and home (or nursing home or other provider), provides and supports self-management education and training, directs communication between patient/caregiver and primary-care provider, and provides intensive follow-up of patient and caregiver following hospital discharge.

5. Establish uniform plan of care and/or transition forms/ checklists for use by your usual transition partners. Providers

need a uniform care plan and standardized protocols for transfers across settings to facilitate communication and continuity. Build consensus around standard practices for select and at-risk populations using more than one setting. Standardized lists of medications and treatments greatly reduce the risk of error and the likelihood of not having needed supplies.

6. Involve emergency medical systems (EMS) or other transport service providers to assist in continuity. Involve local transport providers in your project and have them recognize uniform transfer forms and standardized transfer protocols. Make them responsible for the transfer of advance care plans across settings. In Oregon, for instance, EMS crews are authorized to act on the POLST (the standardized, state-wide advance care planning/advance directive document; see http://www.polst.org) to avoid unwanted interventions.

7. Regionalize electronic medical information transfer. This is designed to facilitate the timely transfer of essential information across settings. Healthcare providers need an accessible medical record that contains current patient information (e.g., problem and medication lists; physical, cognitive, and functional status information; physician and caregiver contact information, etc.). In addition, electronic information transfer can increase patient safety.

8. Create an extended care pathway. These pathways provide protocols for each phase of a patient's care, including the roles that the interdisciplinary clinicians should play. Often, preparation for a patient's transition from one care setting to the next is an explicit element of such protocols.

Tools and Resources

- American Geriatrics Society, Position Statement: Improving the Quality of Transitional Care for Person with Complex Care Needs
  http://www.americangeriatrics.org
- *Merck Manual of Health and Aging*
  http://www.merck.com/pubs/mmanual_ha/contents.html
- The Care Transitions Program and Health Sciences Center at the University of Colorado–Denver
  http://www.care transitions.org
- Medication Reconciliation, Institute for Healthcare Improvement
  http://www.ihi.org/ihi/topics/patientsafety/medication systems/tools/medication+reconciliation+flowsheet.htm
- Joint Commission on Accreditation of Healthcare Organizations, Sentinel Event Alert, No. 35
  http://www.jcaho.org/SentinelEvents/SentinelEventAlert/ sea.htm

8

Chronic Care
Heart and Lung Failure

In This Chapter

- Disease-management strategies
- The role of the family caregiver
- End-of-life issues, such as how to make advance care plans
- Living well with the disease

Chronic organ system failure presents a distinct trajectory of illness, with an erratic and unpredictable course characterized by periods of relative stability punctuated by episodes of severe illness, all set against a background of gradual, progressive disability. Patient needs range from having oxygen reliably available at home to being hospitalized repeatedly. Along the way, family caregivers need support and help, too, with everything from managing medication to navigating Medicare benefits. The current healthcare structure usually offers these patients and families a patchwork of services, although some providers or payers now provide disease management and care coordination.

Cardiovascular and pulmonary diseases are complex. Treatment requires the expertise of medical specialists, rehabilitative therapies, support services, and an array of medications. Helping patients and caregivers understand the disease and its treatment will allow them to better appreciate why they are seeing certain clinicians, why the patient is behaving in certain ways, or why some treatments work and others may not. Talking to patients and their caregivers about what to expect as the illness progresses may help them feel more confident in their ability to manage everything, especially in the home. By talking about advance directives and preferences for care, the family will be prepared to act on the patient's behalf when necessary.

Although heart and lung disease are among the leading causes of death, most families will feel that the death itself was sudden and unexpected, even if the patient had been ill for years. Patients and families tend not to realize that the disease is eventually fatal, usually because no one has discussed this with them directly but also because patients recover from episodes of severe illness and then experience a long period of adequate function within constraints. Death is very unpredictable in these patients and may come suddenly in any of these episodes.

The best approach for serving these patients is to blend palliative care services with the best of medical treatment and disease management. For these patients, clinicians must be committed to pursuing aggressive life-extending treatment while providing comfort care and support in addressing end-of-life concerns and needs. The teams that have worked to improve care have found that they need to provide continuity, coordination, excellent symptom management, advance care planning, maintenance of function, patient/family counseling and support, and attention to spiritual and personal growth.

Our teams found that six areas of care regularly respond to the application of quality improvement (QI) methods: disease and symptom management; coordination and continuity of care; 24/7 crisis management; patient and family education and support for self-management; advance care planning; and patient and family support.

Throughout this chapter, "Team Pulse" represents a composite of work done by various successful teams with whom we have worked (see Chapter 2 for basic methods).

IDENTIFYING THE PROBLEM AND SETTING AN AIM

TEAM PULSE

Team Pulse, based in a veterans' medical center, had more than the usual share of patients with advanced heart or lung disease. They wanted to improve the care that these patients received in the last two or three years of life. Most of all, Team Pulse wanted to reduce the number of 911 calls and unplanned hospital and emergency department (ED) admissions. This desire was just a hunch, based on conversations among doctors and nurses and a sense that patients and caregivers seemed almost battered by repeatedly showing up in the ED and intensive care unit (ICU). Before agreeing to work on this problem, the team decided to gather data, which was relatively straightforward, given the Veterans Health Administration's (VHA) extensive electronic records. It turned out that the hunch was on target: in a review of one year's worth of admissions data, patients with CHF or COPD who were "frequent fliers," were hospitalized much more often than patients with other diseases, and the rates were well above those reported in the professional literature.

Rather than acting on vague ideas, Team Pulse met to discuss what each member had observed about the causes of readmission and ED visits for CHF/COPD patients. They interviewed a few patients and their caregivers to hear about the problems that led them to return to the ED or to be hospitalized. After a few meetings, the team chose the following aim.

Aim: *Within 60 days, advanced CHF/COPD patients will have reduced by 75% 911 calls and unplanned hospital/ED admissions.*

They defined "advanced" as a patient who had been hospitalized within the last six months for an exacerbation, unless the patient could walk for six minutes at the follow-up clinic visit. They added the last criterion because the clinic almost always did this test, and it was more reliably available than ejection fractions or oxygenation levels. Also, it directed attention to the patient's function.

Like Team Pulse, you may see many patients who become overwhelmed by symptoms and end up in the emergency department, with some appearing several times per year. This situation reflects how ill-prepared patients and loved ones are to respond to early warnings when symptoms worsen. Sometimes an exacerbation is the result of an upset in the patient's disease-management routine, such as mismanagement of medications or diet, undue stress, or exercise. Learning to manage these triggers can help.

Your team might want to explore the following issues:

- What is it about the symptom-management protocol that is not working? Can you fix it?
- Are your patients anxious about self-care? Do they need reassurance and education about their condition?
- What are the other issues that you face with this population?

Once you have a clear understanding of problems for your patients, establish an aim statement. Make sure the statement includes the four key components.

Aim: In 60 days, CHF/COPD patients referred to the palliative care program will have reduced the number of 911 calls and unplanned hospital/ED admissions by 75%.

What will improve: The number of 911 calls and unplanned hospital/ED admissions.

By when: Within 60 days.

By how much: Seventy-five percent.

For whom: CHF/COPD patients referred to the palliative care program.

CHOOSING A TEAM

TEAM PULSE

The doctor and nurse who wanted to kick off the QI project knew that the fragmented care being provided to CHF/COPD patients was inadequate. They were sure that they could offer more integrated services to meet patients' needs while simultaneously reducing the burden on healthcare. By setting up a disease education and management program, they could help patients gain the confidence and skills needed to manage illness at home. The next step was to identify colleagues who shared their interests and convictions and would commit to serving one year with the QI project. At first, the two recruited another nurse manager and a discharge planner. Eventually, the team grew to include a cardiologist, a home health aide, a hospice nurse liaison, two case managers, and a social worker.

Successful QI teams always include key players. Our CHF/COPD teams find that they need a physician or nurse practitioner "champion," someone with the clinical expertise and administrative know-how to get the project done. Deciding whom to include on your team requires some thought. It might seem obvious that you would include a cardiologist or pulmonologist, but what about home health nurses, a disease-management expert, or an information technology (IT) person? You do not want to assemble a team so large that you are tied up working on committee organizing, but you do want to have enough people with enough information to get something done.

Your setting will affect the composition of your team. A nursing home team, for instance, might be quite different from a hospice team. Depending on your issues, try to include key people that are involved in the current flow of your processes. We have found that six to eight people is reasonable: with less than that, you may not be able to see and understand the whole process; with more, you will not be able to get the team together. Over time, as your work proves to be successful, invite more people to join your team, or spin off a new team on another nursing unit, for instance, in a different home health agency, or to address another topic.

MEASURING SUCCESS

TEAM PULSE

Team Pulse was sure that its ideas would lead to reduced 911 calls and unplanned admissions. However, to check that they were making an improvement, they needed to collect data over time, both to help them understand the effect of their work and also to help them make a convincing case to senior management. They devised a measurement strategy and collected baseline data before making any changes, and they continued to collect that data to see the effect of their work. The team finally decided to track the following measures.

Process Measure: The percentage of patients and caregivers who said that they felt confident to manage symptoms at home.
Outcome Measures: The number of patients (or caregivers) who called 911; the percentage of patients who had unplanned hospital admissions.

The only way to know whether you reach your aim—and whether it is an improvement—is to measure your work. Measurement allows you to quantify the changes made and determine whether or not a specific change really works. Your measures should answer specific questions about the changes being tested. For example, did any patients attend the new education program? How many patients called the nurse manager each day to report weight changes and other symptoms? How many caregivers called 911? What triggered the call?

Following are some examples of measures to use with advanced CHF/COPD QI efforts (see Chapter 2 for basic information about measures).

Process Measures

- Patients and caregivers who participate in education programs or disease-management programs.
- Calls to the nurse practitioner.
- Patients who receive 24-hour nursing support.
- Patients' and caregivers' awareness of danger symptoms before and after education sessions.
- Number of times that patients managed danger symptoms at home after initial training and a phone call with a nurse or physician.

Outcome Measures

- Proportion of unplanned hospitalizations.
- Number of emergency department (ED) visits.
- Number of 911 calls.
- Patients and caregivers who felt confident managing symptoms at home.
- Patients who have clear advance care plans, including treatment decisions regarding time-limited trials, sedation, and intubation.
- Smoking cessation.
- Hospital or ED length of stay.

Adverse-Effect Measures

- Patients who receive a wrong dose of medication at home.
- Management of side effects of medications at home.

You want to track one or two key indicators over time and collect just enough data to convince a benevolent skeptic. (And that skeptic is usually yourself!) Remember, you are not conducting medical research; you need data that are credible and on target but not extensive. If you are trying to find out how many patients with advanced CHF/COPD called 911 despite the education program, you need that data (and perhaps their presenting symptoms). You do not need much else.

Another issue to consider when planning your measurement strategy is to get a manageable data size. If there are too few patients, then you need to roll up a longer time or review whether this change is really a priority for your institution. With too few patients, you might just adopt best practices from elsewhere and not focus on QI as the method for change. If you have an abundance of patients, then you need to have a sampling plan to get unbiased data. The sampling can aim for simplicity: for example, the first week's discharges each month.

TELLING YOUR STORY: TIME SERIES GRAPH

Many teams find that they can make the most convincing case about the improvement made (or the need for improvement) by presenting data in a time series chart. First, decide which data to collect and how often, and confirm who will be responsible for collecting it. You can then decide whether to collect data daily, weekly, monthly, or quarterly. The numbers of patients and the nature of the change you are testing will drive the frequency of collection; you want to collect enough data to be able to see what is happening. So, if you decide to look at 911 calls, you might have enough call volume to collect this weekly; if not, try it monthly. Patient participation in education programs might be worth collecting monthly, while the number of patients calling in to report weight fluctuation and other symptoms could probably be collected weekly.

TEAM PULSE

To measure its progress, Team Pulse decided to chart three changes: the proportion of patients and caregivers who felt confident in managing symptoms at home, based on a self-administered survey at their outpatient clinic visit; the percentage of patients who had unplanned hospital or ED admissions each month; and the number of 911 calls each month. Some of the results that Team Pulse tracked on the time series charts are given in Figures 8.1 and 8.2.

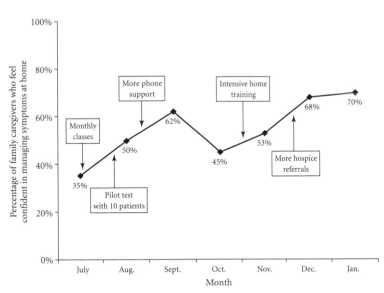

FIGURE 8.1 Family caregivers' confidence levels

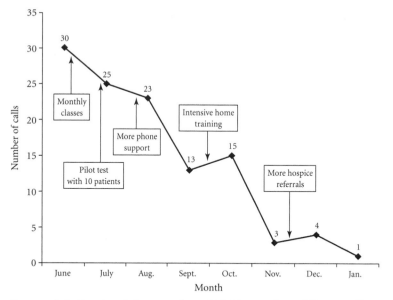

FIGURE 8.2 Caregivers' distress calls to 911. The number of distress calls made by hospice patients at home decreased during the test period.

IDENTIFYING AND TESTING CHANGES

TEAM PULSE

Team Pulse came up with a list of ideas that could reduce 911 calls and unplanned hospital admissions. They decided which interventions to test and chose a small initial sample. They tested each intervention by starting with 10 patients and caregivers and with a team that included a physician and two nurses. This small group participated in four training sessions to learn about managing disease at home. They also received an at-home "911 kit" for emergencies, which came with the understanding that a home-care nurse would come to the house whenever possible or that a nurse would walk them through a crisis by phone. After three months, in which none of the patients was readmitted, the team expanded the program to another 10 patients. They continued to monitor the original 10 for hospital readmissions. Once they were able to see improvement, they applied the interventions on a broader scale.

In ordinary Medicare practice, there is so much room for improvement in caring for CHF/COPD patients in their final years of life that your team will certainly find a place to start. Care for patients at all stages of advanced heart and lung disease should be based on concepts of disease management. Their care should include coordinated healthcare interventions along with communications regarding patient self-care. A CHF/COPD disease-management protocol should do the following.

- Support the clinician–patient relationship and plan of care.
- Emphasize prevention of disease-related exacerbations and complications using evidence-based guidelines.
- Monitor weight, function, and symptoms everyday, and start appropriate treatment right away.
- Use patient-empowerment tools to help patients manage at home.
- Evaluate outcomes on an ongoing basis with the goal of improving overall health.
- Improve patients' access to services, including immunization and prescription drugs.

Try a few ideas from this list based on what we have learned working with teams around the country.

Change Ideas for Better CHF/COPD Management

- Provide patients with ready access, around-the-clock, to a nurse care manager, and improve patient–provider communication, especially via telephone.
- Offer quick assessment and treatment of symptoms.

- Establish community-based care-management protocols with primary care doctors so that nurses can manage patients at home without the usual restrictions of home healthcare.
- Establish comfort care protocols for CHF and COPD patients; these protocols should reflect the patient's stage of life. For example, one protocol should reflect the needs of patients who have lived with the disease for a short time; another could reflect the needs of patients likely to die within a year.
- Refer appropriate patients to hospice, and work with a hospice program to be sure that its services are appropriate. Hospice can provide 24/7 support, but patients are still able to get medical interventions (including being on waiting lists for transplants).
- Set up monthly education and group support programs for caregivers and for patients well enough to accompany them. These sessions should give caregivers practical information on issues such as how to recognize danger signs, the importance of advance care plans, when to call the case-management nurse, and so on.
- Create a 911 kit for home use with medications to treat dyspnea, pain, and other distressing symptoms. Family members should be confident that they know how to use the kit, and the kit can be available in the home for the on-call nurse to provide instructions.

Common Barriers to Good CHF/COPD Management

TEAM PULSE

As the project expanded, the team was disappointed to discover that caregivers were still reluctant to manage some symptoms at home, es-

pecially symptoms that involved breathing problems. Caregivers found that these were just too scary and that their own confidence was too shaky. To counter this, the team enhanced its training sessions. In addition to the education session, a home-care nurse visited each patient and family four times over the course of one month to discuss symptoms, review treatment, and provide support. This intervention really seemed to boost caregivers' confidence. The team found that intense work in the early days following discharge was more effective than using a prolonged education process. They also started referring appropriate patients to hospice, since that guaranteed 24/7 at-home coverage. However, they did find that the hospice nurses and physicians needed training and back-up on optimal medical treatment for these complex patients.

While our case and explanation here have focused on good disease management, self-care, and rapid response, another important issue often confounds good care for CHF and COPD patients: the challenge of planning for dying when the prognosis stays ambiguous. No matter how limited their heart and lungs, if they are stable, these patients might live for many months, or even years—or they might die tomorrow. It is as if they are skating on very thin ice, but no one can know just how it will break or if a rescue will work. So dying often seems sudden, even though it was likely for many months.

Think back to the characterization of "dying or not" in Chapter 1. Our practices with regard to advance care planning, hospice eligibility, family farewells, and spiritual peace all start with the dying person. But CHF and COPD patients live with the constant risk of dying. In order to plan ahead, we need better practices and ways of thinking.

Our QI teams regularly make major gains by counseling every patient about the need to plan for the chance of sudden dying: we call it "contingency planning," or "planning for the worst and hoping for the best." Somehow, patients and others think that it is only acceptable to get their lives in order and say farewells once. The palliative care team (or primary-care nurse or doctor) has to give the patient permission to attend to issues of life closure, with the chance that he or she will live long enough to have to do it again.

Once the team is over this hurdle, advance care planning for serious COPD and CHF patients usually grows to 80–90% within one or two months. And making plans for time-limited trials on the ventilator and for sedation near death make it more likely that those things will happen, without the burdens created when such plans go unmade.

With modern-day complexities in healthcare situations, as you work toward your goal, you will encounter some barriers. Anticipating and preparing for them will allow your team to overcome problems while staying focused on its aim. Some of the common barriers that CHF/COPD teams face are the following.

- Hospitals and specialists may not welcome reduced hospitalizations; you may have to make a convincing case for professional ethics and mission while watching for any other advantages.
- Inadequate clinical information systems.
- Lack of knowledge or awareness about the merits of disease management.
- Referrals to hospice or palliative care for patients who do not seem to be "dying."

GIVE THEM SOMETHING TO TALK ABOUT

TEAM PULSE

By the end of the first year, Team Pulse had learned a lot about managing CHF/COPD patients during the final stages of life. In these cases, they discovered that families needed very intense support with lots of in-person involvement from a nurse and, sometimes, the physician. They were able to convince their senior administrators about the advantages of their program and received more funding to continue and build on their current efforts. Indeed, they expanded to other parts of the organization. Eventually, the team realized that it might be able to enhance its partnership with the hospice program. Hospitalizations were halved and 911 calls were rare.

TOOLS AND RESOURCES

Admission Orders: Hope Hospice developed an example of a good admission order, which can be found online at http://www .mywhatever.com/cifwriter/content/66/4412.html or in J. Lynn, J. L. Schuster, and A. Kabcenell's *Improving Care for the End of Life: A Sourcebook for Clinicians and Managers.*

Home Comfort Kit: Several teams have developed cardiac-care comfort kits that help patients to manage symptoms at home. These kits include the full range of medication that a cardiac patient might need to ensure that patients and caregivers can readily handle crises as they occur. Some of the medications that are in the kits for CHF patients developed by Hope Hospice are:

- Nitroglycerin 0.4 mg (1 bottle)
- Morphine 10mg/5cc UD #2
- Morphine inject 10mg #2
- Furosemide 40 mg #4
- Furosemide 100 mg IV #2
- IV/subc access kit
- Lorazepam 0.5 mg #5
- Naproxen 500 mg #2

- Sucralfate 1 gm/10 cc #2
- Maalox Plus 30 ml UD #2
- Normal saline 2.5 ml UD #4
- Compazine 10 mg po #2
- Compazine 25 mg PR #2
- ASA 325 mg #1
- Pentobarbital supp 60 mg #4

Caregiver support: free workbook guides for both CHF and
COPD at http://www.medicaring.org

NURSING HOME QUALITY
Pressure Ulcers

IN THIS CHAPTER

- Preventing and healing pressure ulcers
- Making improvement work in nursing homes

Among the many fears that old and frail people have, none is as distressing and immediate as that of developing a bedsore, a serious pressure ulcer. These lesions cause pain, limit mobility, alter self-image and relationships, and add substantially to costs. Although pressure ulcers often arise in hospitals or in home care, they are a special burden and threat among residents in nursing homes. This chapter focuses on QI strategies that work in nursing home environments. The information about preventing and treating pressure ulcers can be applied in other settings as well.

TEAM SPRINGFIELD

A few nurses at Springfield Nursing Home were talking before morning rounds after a particularly difficult week—the surveyors had been there, they had weathered a snowstorm, and the interim director of nursing was moving on to a new job before her successor had been hired. They all felt beaten down, but one nurse said, "Nothing gets to me like the pressure ulcers. I have two new Stage II patients after the weekend, and I can't seem to get any progress on the three I've been working on for months." Another nurse said, "You know, the nursing home I worked in last year has really focused on this, and they are getting down to almost none. Why don't we learn what they are doing and just get it underway? We don't have to wait for things to settle down. If we do, we'll never get started." The unit nurses rallied and got the executive director to agree to explore possible changes on that very same day. After all, one of the deficiencies that the director was facing was that the nursing home was not doing enough quality improvement.

IDENTIFYING THE PROBLEM AND SETTING AN AIM

Good care for pressure ulcers builds on two goals:

1. prevent every lesion you can;
2. heal those that still occur.

Eventually, most teams that take on pressure ulcers work with both issues, but one is probably more important or promising than the other at the outset in each setting. To figure out where to start, consider the following questions:

- Does your facility have a regular and reliable way to assess risk?
- Does your staff implement prevention strategies right away for high-risk residents?
- Does your facility have a higher or lower than average rate of pressure ulcers in high-risk and low-risk residents on Nursing Home Compare?
- Do Stage II ulcers generally heal within two weeks?
- Does your staff have a way to routinely follow indicators of healing on Stage III and IV ulcers?
- Does your facility ensure close attention to any situation in which there is no healing after a few weeks?

If you find that major opportunities for improvement are in the first three items listed, tackle prevention first. If the opportunities are in the last three, tackle healing first. Either way, do it all within a year. Be able to promise residents and families that they will have the very best prevention and healing for this dreaded complication of disability and frailty.

And remember, assessing the opportunities for improvement is likely to highlight the gap between present practices and good performance—but this is what you *aim* to fix. And as you get started, you need to have the commitment of staff and leadership. Setting initial *aims* often requires input from staff, residents, families, and perhaps licensure and certification reviewers. Be prepared to ask others what they think should be done.

TEAM SPRINGFIELD

The Springfield Nursing Home team knew that settling on an aim was central to their success, but they were torn between tackling the pressure ulcers that they were already treating and preventing new ones. After some discussion, they decided first to eradicate new ones, even while paying more attention to those chronic, nonhealing ones. This discussion started in early August, and the executive director suggested that they plan to have the problem under control within one year. Someone else said, "We'd better have it down solid before next summer—we are always juggling around vacations and staff changes in July and August. Let's aim to get this project in place before June." Then another nurse raised the stakes, saying, "You know, I can't face coming in to find one more pressure ulcer! I know it will take more than a few weeks, but why can't we promise one another to have at least the new-onset pressure ulcers under control within a few months?" Thus, the team ended up with the following initial aim.

Aim: *Within 30 days, Springfield Nursing Home will have no new Stage II, III, or IV pressure ulcers arising within the facility.*

> **What will improve:** *Occurrence of new Stage II, III, or IV pressure ulcers.*
>
> **By when:** *Within 30 days.*
>
> **By how much:** *One hundred percent improvement, no new pressure ulcers.*
>
> **For whom:** *Residents at Springfield Nursing Home.*

Quality improvement always requires clear and effective aims that are important, measurable, time-limited, and bold. Here are some examples to inspire you.

Sample Prevention Aims

Aim 1: Within one month, residents of your nursing facility will have *no new pressure ulcers.*

Aim 2: Within a month, *every interdisciplinary team meeting will document* each resident's risk for pressure ulcers and review the adequacy of care plans to prevent onset.

Aim 3: Within *six months, every* resident at increased risk for pressure ulcers will be using an appropriate *pressure-reducing* mattress and seating surface.

Aim 4: Within *six months, all resident transfers* to and from the hospital will ensure care within care plan parameters for safety regarding the risk of causing pressure ulcers.

Sample Wound Healing Aims

Aim 1: Within two months, *all* Stage II pressure ulcers will be *healed* within three weeks of onset.

Aim 2: Within six months, *all* Stage III and IV pressure ulcers *that do not show healing* within three weeks *will have a change of plan,* and all that do not show healing within six weeks will have *wound care consultation.*

Aim 3: Within three months, all routine wound care will be *converted to one of four treatment protocols;* exceptions will be clearly *documented* as to rationale and time limits; and errors in implementation of wound care protocols will be *eliminated.*

Some Pointers to Remember as You Build Your Aim

- *Some facilities really can aim for no new-onset pressure ulcers.* If you attempt this goal, you may need to come up with a more precise aim, one that excludes people who are very close to death (when even turning the person can become irrelevant, and skin is sometimes tissue-paper fragile). You might even have to exempt residents who take imprudent risks, despite good counseling. But often, you really can drive the rate of onsite onset very low. If you have a very difficult population or situation, you might instead have to *aim* to cut your current rate in half or to get under the national average.
- *The opportunities for error are enormous.* Missing just one turning out of 1,000 will yield two periods of exposure to prolonged ischemia each year for each resident. The reliability of prevention requires the level of performance required of airplane pilots. The only way to achieve this is with routinization of the prevention practices, applying a high priority to the work, and tolerating redundant work at critical junctures.
- *Assessment matters: early and often!* You have to know not only that a particular resident is at high risk but also the cause of that risk. The interventions to reduce risk have to be matched to the origins of risk.
- *Very high performing facilities end up reaching out* to their hospitals, home care, and emergency services; otherwise, their residents get skin damage in these affiliated settings. Think

about whether your *aim* requires some partners from other organizations.

- *Unless the resident is close to death, wounds should heal, even if slowly.* Many of our teams found that simply overcoming complacency about the treatment (viewing pressure ulcers as an inevitable part of being very frail and approaching the end of life rather than seeing it as a preventable and treatable condition) allowed substantial healing.

- *Stage I lesions indicate high risk* and the need for *changes* in the care plan; Stage II lesions are worth tallying but still mainly point to risk and the need for changes in the care plan; but Stage III and IV lesions are miserable. Eradicating them is the real goal, no matter what shorter-term and more common *aim* you target.

- *Convergence on a small set of protocols* for assessment, prevention, and treatment allows major leaps forward in quality. The nursing staff cannot become experts in dozens of approaches that seem to have no rationale beyond the current interests or worries of the attending physician or head nurse.

You will notice that some of the aims focus on process and others focus on outcomes. If you have a major problem with pressure ulcers and you are in a large facility, you will have enough wounds to monitor. However, many facilities have smaller numbers of ulcers or residents (or both), and just tracking pressure ulcer onset or healing will not be enough; the small numbers will not allow you to know whether your team is really getting better or whether it just happens to be a good month. In that case, monitoring the process is often better, since correct procedures apply to every resident (for prevention) or every wound (for healing).

In general, the time frames for prevention can be short, usually within a few months at most. However, the time frames for improving healing can take longer, since the rate of healing is often slow in nursing home residents, even with optimal care.

Choosing a Team

Team Springfield

The Springfield project began with unit head nurses and the blessing of the executive director. At their first lunchtime meeting, the group realized that none of them had any formal training in quality improvement (QI) and no special expertise in wound prevention, though they all had practical experience in both arenas. One team member said that she would try to persuade her friend, who had led successful reforms in a neighboring facility, to talk to their group: "She will be delighted to share all they learned; let me see how to get her over here." The new director of nursing, who had decided to sit in on the meeting, offered to check with the local quality improvement organization (QIO) to see if it would help with quality improvement training. Then another nurse said, "You know, my lead CNA is really good at this work, and she's been here for years. She's pretty concerned with the recent spate of new-onset ulcers, and the other CNAs respect her. Let's invite her to join our team." The ensuing discussion also highlighted the benefit of involving the nurse who did preadmission assessments, since she might start working with ambulances and transfers.

Who needs to be part of your team? Many of our nursing home teams have found the strongest leadership and commitment among their direct care workers, especially LPNs and CNAs. Be sure your team leaders include staff members, especially those who turn the patients, give the baths, and suffer with the residents when a pressure ulcer arises. Someone on your team has to be a real expert on pressure ulcer prevention and wound treatment. Some teams have sent a nurse or two off for wound care training, some have hired a consultant, and some have picked up those skills with self-education onsite. Once the nursing home has developed this expertise, it may be of value to local hospitals and home care agencies, and consultation among them often results in many good spin-offs in terms of coordinating best practices.

As always, someone on the team has to take charge of the QI process: scheduling meetings, setting plans, monitoring data, and aggressively implementing improvements. To succeed, the team needs support from the facility's administrative leadership. The federal government requires that nursing homes engage in QI, and rates of pressure ulcers are publicly reported, so senior leadership should support your work and trumpet your success.

Since pressure ulcer prevention and healing have been major focuses of Medicare, substantial resources to help you with measurement and changes are readily available at http://www.medqic.org. Have a look, and use their instruments, brochures, and pointers.

Measuring Success

Team Springfield

Team Springfield settled on taking responsibility for every new-onset Stage II, III, or IV lesion that happened to one of their residents, even if it happened while the resident was out with family, off to see a physician, or being transferred to or from a hospital. Using an existing reporting method, they tallied the lesions reported in the previous month, finding that they had 22 new Stage II lesions and two Stage III and IV lesions. Stage III and IV lesions really cause suffering for patients; Stage II wounds reflect breakdowns in care technique. Because there were so many Stage II lesions, the group decided to track them separately from other lesions. The team felt that any new Stage III or IV wound was calamitous and would require a lot of soul-searching and review. They knew that a few Stage II blisters might not really be avoidable, but they did not want to be complacent.

The group could not at first decide how to report its results. There was some discussion about how to calculate the percentage of patients who developed pressure ulcers, but the team decided that since they were going for zero occurrences, percentages did not really matter. Instead, the group decided to count absolute numbers of lesions with the aim of eventually having none. The team agreed to tally the results each month.

Below are some measurement strategies to track your progress.

For Prevention of Pressure Ulcers

- New admissions with Braden Score risk assessment within four hours of arrival (or before).
- All residents with medium or high risk scores addressed at each interdisciplinary team meeting.
- Residents at high risk who are using appropriate pressure-reducing surfaces on beds and chairs.
- Residents with daily skin inspection.
- Residents whose possible Stage I lesions receive attention with a change in their care plans within the nursing shift when a Stage I lesion is found.
- Time between new onset of Stage III or IV pressure ulcers in the facility.

- Residents with any new-onset Stage II, III, or IV pressure ulcers.
- Admissions or new admissions who had new-onset lesions.

For Healing Pressure Ulcers

- Residents with a Stage II pressure ulcer that healed within three weeks of onset.
- Weekly pressure ulcer evaluations that show measurable improvement since the previous week.
- Residents whose worst pressure ulcer shows measurable improvement each month.
- Pressure ulcers showing no improvement in three weeks which have a change in treatment protocol.
- Pressure ulcers showing no improvement in six weeks which have wound care consultation.

Tools for Measuring Lesions

The best available tool for measuring lesions is probably the Pressure Ulcer Scale for Healing (PUSH) Scale, available at http://www.npuap .org/push3–0.html. Its major limitation is that it does not actually extend to large lesions. You can make a reasonable accommodation simply by measuring (in centimeters) the largest opening of the skin for each pressure ulcer and the dimension at right angles, then multiplying those, and counting the result as an index of the surface area affected. That turns out to be fairly sensitive to healing. So, a pressure ulcer that is 10 cm across at its largest length and 5 cm across at its widest is indexed as $5 \times 10 = 50$ cm². The opening is not really rectangular, of course, but the point is that healing will show in length and width, so the centimeter-squared score will show improvement.

Try using the PUSH Tool below. It is available for download from the National Pressure Ulcer Advisory Panel Web site at http://www .npuap.org/PDF/push3.pdf.

Pressure Ulcer Scale for Healing (PUSH)
PUSH Tool 3.0

Patient Name_____ Patient ID# _____

Ulcer Location _____ Date _____

Directions:

Observe and measure the pressure ulcer. Categorize the ulcer with respect to surface area, exudate, and type of wound tissue. Record a sub-score for each of these ulcer characteristics. Add the sub-scores to obtain the total score. A comparison of total scores measured over time provides an indication of the improvement or deterioration in pressure ulcer healing.

	0	1	2	3	4	5	Sub-score
LENGTH X WIDTH	0	< 0.3	0.3 – 0.6	0.7 – 1.0	1.1 – 2.0	2.1 – 3.0	
	6	**7**	**8**	**9**	**10**		
(in cm²)		3.1 – 4.0	4.1 – 8.0	8.1 – 12.0	12.1 – 24.0	> 24.0	
EXUDATE AMOUNT	**0** None	**1** Light	**2** Moderate	**3** Heavy			Sub-score
TISSUE TYPE	**0** Closed	**1** Epithelial Tissue	**2** Granulation Tissue	**3** Slough	**4** Necrotic Tissue		Sub-score
							TOTAL SCORE

Length x Width: Measure the greatest length (head to toe) and the greatest width (side to side) using a centimeter ruler. Multiply these two measurements (length x width) to obtain an estimate of surface area in square centimeters (cm²). Caveat: Do not guess! Always use a centimeter ruler and always use the same method each time the ulcer is measured.

Exudate Amount: Estimate the amount of exudate (drainage) present after removal of the dressing and before applying any topical agent to the ulcer. Estimate the exudate (drainage) as none, light, moderate, or heavy.

Tissue Type: This refers to the types of tissue that are present in the wound (ulcer) bed. Score as a "4" if there is any necrotic tissue present. Score as a "3" if there is any amount of slough present and necrotic tissue is absent. Score as a "2" if the wound is clean and contains granulation tissue. A superficial wound that is reepithelializing is scored as a "1". When the wound is closed, score as a "0".

4 – **Necrotic Tissue (Eschar):** black, brown, or tan tissue that adheres firmly to the wound bed or ulcer edges and may be either firmer or softer than surrounding skin.

3 – **Slough:** yellow or white tissue that adheres to the ulcer bed in strings or thick clumps, or is mucinous.

2 – **Granulation Tissue:** pink or beefy red tissue with a shiny, moist, granular appearance.

1 – **Epithelial Tissue:** for superficial ulcers, new pink or shiny tissue (skin) that grows in from the edges or as islands on the ulcer surface.

0 – **Closed/Resurfaced:** the wound is completely covered with epithelium (new skin).

Pressure Ulcer Healing Chart
To monitor trends in PUSH Scores over time
(Use a separate page for each pressure ulcer)

Patient Name_____ Patient ID# _____

Ulcer Location _____ Date _____

Directions:
Observe and measure pressure ulcers at regular intervals using the PUSH Tool.
Date and record PUSH Sub-scores and Total Scores on the Pressure Ulcer Healing Record below.

Pressure Ulcer Healing **Record**													
Date													
Length x Width													
Exudate Amount													
Tissue Type													
PUSH Total Score													

Graph the PUSH Total Scores on the Pressure Ulcer Healing Graph below.

PUSH Total Score	Pressure Ulcer Healing **Graph**												
17													
16													
15													
14													
13													
12													
11													
10													
9													
8													
7													
6													
5													
4													
3													
2													
1													
Healed = 0													
Date													

PUSH Tool Version 3.0: 9/15/98
©National Pressure Ulcer Advisory Panel

Telling Your Story: Time Series Graph

Once you have begun tracking data, you will want a way to display it so as to tell the story of your progress (or note the other interventions you have tried when one did not work out). Details on how to chart results are included in Chapter 2. Figure 9.1 shows how charts can be used to dramatically illustrate change and improvement.

Identifying and Testing Changes

Team Springfield

Team Springfield found that its first set of interventions was just to get the nursing home's current practices up to the team's own protocols.

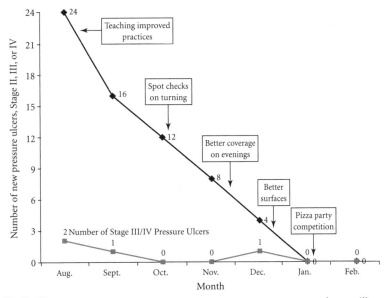

Figure 9.1 Within 30 days, no new Stage II, III, or IV pressure ulcers will arise within the facility

The team launched in-service training for all direct care staff, ensured that the admissions forms for risk assessment were done on time, and made sure that the current system of turning and repositioning patients was followed. Then the two CNAs on the team volunteered to do some spot-checking on high-risk patients and report back. The reports were daunting: nearly half of the needed turnings were not done on time on the evening shift, especially during supper. It took time to rearrange the feeding schedule and to get an extra turning team on the evening shift, but it worked.

The team started tracking every pressure lesion, including Stage I lesions. The team found that the residents needed better sitting surfaces, that the facility needed more pressure-relieving mattresses, and that a few residents were getting skin lesions from disposable diapers at night. Team members whittled away at all of these problems. They got the facility to give CNAs prizes and recognition for reporting Stage I lesions. They trained all staff and regular volunteers on how to help shift residents' sitting positions and how to recognize that this was needed. They had most new admissions receiving risk assessment with the Braden Score even before admission and always within the first few hours. The nurse getting the extra training brought back many ideas and success stories. The QIO helped with checking on the measurement and graphing the results, which were displayed prominently in the employee dining room.

Eventually, the team started working much more with their ambulance and transport service and their local hospital, since it gradually became clear that improving procedures just within their own walls was not going to protect their residents well enough. Their tally in September did not show much gain, just a few less Stage II lesions and only one Stage III lesion. But October came and went without any Stage III or IV wounds and with only half as many Stage II ulcers. By the end of November, units were in a sort of informal competition to see how long they could go into the month before they saw any Stage II lesions, and the month ended with just eight Stage II lesions (compared with 22 when they started) and no onsite Stage III or IV wounds. Everyone felt much better about work, and observers started noting that family meetings were much smoother when the staff could promise to prevent pressure ulcers. The remaining ulcers were quickly healed, and new ones tended to occur either in residents who were capable of refusing to go along with the recommended treatment and did so or in residents who were just starting to get very sick. The nurses realized that these groups and those coming from outside the facility were going to require some further work.

Most of what works in pressure ulcer prevention and treatment is, simply, *good care*—given over and over, and reliably. There are all sorts of fads for costly mattresses, high-tech diagnostic tests, and costly dressings. None of these, however, has good evidence behind it. Be very cautious of an eager salesperson offering to solve your pressure ulcer problems with some costly technological fix. Most of these divert attention from the core issues: reliable assessment, frequent repositioning, and aggressive wound care.

What Are Some Things That I Can Try to Improve Healing in My Facility?

- Hold weekly interdisciplinary wound rounds that include nursing assistants.
- Provide consistent access to wound care expertise through advanced training of designated staff and the use of area experts.
- Provide centimeter rulers, calculators, and training to measure length, or use the entire PUSH Tool.
- Monitor healing every week.
- Change treatment plans for nonhealing wounds (with no decrease in PUSH score in two or three weeks).
- Standardize protocols and supplies for the most common types of wounds.

- Establish blame-free peer-to-peer relationships with wound care staff in other healthcare organizations (hospitals, nursing homes, home health agencies).
- Share educational events and wound rounds.
- Conduct shared case reviews of interfacility pressure ulcers.
- Share experts and wound care and transfer protocols.

What Are Some Things That I Can Do to Prevent the Formation of Pressure Ulcers for My Residents?

- Assess risk at admission (within a few hours), with every change in status, and at least quarterly.
- Inspect all of the skin daily, except perhaps in very low-risk residents who find this offensive.
- Encourage direct care staff to report any lesion, potential lesion, or risky situation.
- Give rewards to staff for reporting wounds (e.g., a coupon for credit in the cafeteria).
- Post time series graphs, both by unit and for the entire facility.
- Incorporate pressure ulcer education in new employees' orientation and in annual skills evaluations.
- Highlight resident-specific risk factors and interventions in interfacility transfer forms.
- Give feedback to transferring organizations on all pressure ulcers identified at admission.
- Use local QIO staff to serve as conveners and facilitators of interorganizational efforts to coordinate and improve pressure ulcer care in your community.
- Involve nursing assistants, family members, and residents in the improvement activities.
- Conduct an inquiry for "root causes" for any facility-acquired pressure ulcer, and assess what might have prevented it.

- Identify residents at high risk for pressure ulcers by placing a visual cue at their bedsides.
- Monitor timeliness of repositioning by regular auditing of a random sample of at-risk residents: the auditor places a card with the time of repositioning under selected residents; the card is returned to the auditor at the time of the next repositioning.

GIVE THEM SOMETHING TO TALK ABOUT

TEAM SPRINGFIELD

Team Springfield realized that they were up against the coming holidays and the traditional juggling of vacations and illnesses in midwinter. They were worried that they would lose ground, but they had put in place various steps to guard against that. They had funding for the "turning team," and CNAs enjoyed doing that so much that it was staffed through the holidays. The admissions package, with its risk assessment, was regularly done. The team had no breakdowns in assessment and turning for many weeks. They decided to make it a special competition over the holidays and got a local pizza parlor to donate a pizza party to every unit that managed to get from December 15 to January 15 with no new pressure ulcers. That was just creative enough to get lots of cooperation—and lots of pizza.

Team Springfield came to be a bit of a mythic story in the area, and staff members were invited to share their work with other teams. The QIO had them present their work at a regional conference, and the local newspaper picked it up. The management was a bit concerned about whether it might seem to be adverse publicity to admit that they had been doing so badly just a few months earlier, but a

> *conversation with the reporter convinced the executive director that the story would be sympathetic and generally helpful to the facility's reputation. The good reputation led to the team leader being invited to do training sessions at the local hospital, with the aim of helping to reduce pressure ulcers in its elderly and frail residents. Perhaps most important, the success in stopping onset led the team to concentrate more on healing their chronic ulcers, with similarly good outcomes. Even staff turnover declined.*

Winning the battle against pressure ulcers is good news, so share it! Make sure that other facilities in your area get to learn from your good work. Sometimes teams are reluctant to share insights with other competing facilities in their area. This sentiment is well worth overcoming. No one gains by having some facilities functioning badly, since they harm the general level of staff expertise, hurt residents, let hospitals and ambulances perpetuate inadequate practices, and give nursing homes a bad reputation. Compete on other issues, but help one another to ensure that every resident has the best chance to avoid pressure ulcers.

When you learn some new twist that really helps you succeed, share that with your state QIO, and ask them to put it on http://www.med qic.org. Consider publishing your work in professional and management journals. In one of our projects, the average nursing home participating in a QI collaborative with their local QIO managed to inform more than 100 other facilities.

TOOLS AND RESOURCES

- PUSH Tool for monitoring pressure ulcers
  http://www.npuap .org/PDF/push3.pdf
- Braden Scale for predicting pressure ulcers
  http://www.bradenscale.com

- National Pressure Ulcer Advisory Panel
  http://www.npuap.org/
- Agency for Healthcare Policy and Research
  http://www.ahcpr.gov/clinic/cpgonline.htm
- Medicare Quality Improvement Community
  http://www.medqic.org

10

IMPROVING CARE FOR PEOPLE WITH ADVANCED DEMENTIA AND THEIR FAMILIES

IN THIS CHAPTER

- Recognizing when patients are near the end of life
- Evaluating symptoms in nonverbal patients
- Making improvements work in hospice, residential facilities, adult daycare, and at home

You can recognize people with advanced dementia when you see them. They only say a few words, although some may speak incoherently; they are unable to walk or maintain bowel or bladder control; they may appear either blissfully unaware of their surroundings or anxious, fidgety, restless, or aggravated. Recognizing their needs is harder. Can you promise to provide supportive, comprehensive care to these patients and their loved ones? Do you know how to improve current practices?

This chapter focuses on quality improvement (QI) strategies that work for people with advanced dementias and their families across care settings. This chapter provides information about symptom recognition and management and about caring for the caregiver during the final phase of illness and through bereavement.

TEAM SUNSHINE

The Friendly Family Adult Day Center cared specifically for people with dementia while their caregivers worked or just took a break. The center recently divided its activity programs into two levels: one for those with higher cognitive and physical functioning and one for those with advanced dementia. Were it not for the determination of their family caregivers to keep these patients at home while relying on the center for respite, many clients would have to move to nursing homes.

Splitting into two groups made a difference in the energy, enthusiasm, and participation of the higher functioning group, but the staff questioned whether it benefited those patients with advanced dementia in the "Sunshine Club." The staff member who led the activities and caregiving for the Sunshine Club told the center director, "We need some help. When I see these people all together like this, it reminds me of a bad nursing home. We have a great program for the higher functioning folks, and we've got to do more for those who are worse off."

The director agreed and called the Alzheimer's Association's local chapter, which had considerable experience with families and patients with advanced dementia. They agreed to meet with staff after work.

IDENTIFYING THE PROBLEM AND SETTING AN AIM

When a person with dementia dies, you hope that their family members can look back and say the following:

- Mom did not suffer.
- She lived as fully as possible until death.
- We treated her as a person until the end.
- We had the help that we needed to get through Dad's last phase of life.
- We had the help that we needed working through our grief.
- We were not surprised by things that happened.
- We made the right—or best—choices on treatment decisions.
- We participated in Dad's care in the manner that we wanted.

Although these are goals that healthcare professionals want to achieve for all people in the last phase of life, trying to do so for people with dementia and their families is especially challenging. The nature and length of the illness can make it harder than ever to keep promises or to design meaningful programs. Even so, four areas are ripe for QI, no matter where you work:

- recognizing and relieving discomfort;
- providing appropriate human contact: touch as well as emotional, spiritual, and physical comfort;
- providing supportive services focused on the changing needs of the patient and family;
- avoiding unnecessary hospitalizations, nonbeneficial antibiotic treatment, artificial feeding and hydration, invasive medical tests that will not change the course of the illness, and any unnecessary burden for the family.

Although you may want to tackle everything at once, try to focus on one area, either because it represents a major problem for patients or because it is a problem that you know you can solve. Once you have made improvements in one area, begin working on others. As your team and organization begin to see the results, other staff memebers will join you on the journey to quality care.

Here are some questions to help you get started.

- Are procedures in place to measure symptoms and assess comfort, using tools specific to people with dementia?
- Do staff and family members call patients by name and include references to family members, or other personal history, while giving care?
- Are people with dementia sitting for long periods between meals with no interaction or sensory stimulation?

- Are paid caregivers or family members complaining of getting hurt while caring for patients with advanced dementia?
- Are education and support opportunities for families available for the tough decisions which they will have to make?
- Do you routinely cover treatment decisions and advanced care planning in family meetings?
- Do family members complain that "nobody cares" or that the loved one is not getting the care that is needed?
- Are family members reporting that they are getting too tired to continue, that they do not know what to do for the patient, or that they have no time for themselves?

Review these questions and pick a problem area that has the greatest possibility for improvement. If all these areas need improvement, then start with aims focused on patient care, and then move on from there.

TEAM SUNSHINE

The Sunshine Club staff did not like hearing some of the participants calling out and were uneasy seeing their clients sitting and sleeping in chairs unless they were being assisted with eating or toileting. Thus, they decided to focus on comfort aims. The director agreed that the team should solve this problem first but wanted to start with a group of one dozen clients. If the team tried to fix everything at once, they could be overwhelmed. The team had the right expertise to tackle this project but would need to involve a person knowledgeable about the advanced stages of Alzheimer's disease, a QI specialist, and at least one family member to provide support and ideas. The four-member team chose an initial aim.

Aim: In five months, Sunshine Club participants will have human contact and engagement between meals when observed at regularly scheduled monitoring times at least 90% of the time.

What will improve: *The percentage of times during the day in which people with advanced dementia are observed receiving human contact or engaging in positive activities.*

By how much: *Ninety percent.*

By when: *Within five months.*

For whom: *Members of the Sunshine Club (people with advanced dementia).*

An aim should be clearly stated and measurable; it should address a problem that affects your patients' quality of life. Here are some aims that other teams have used.

Aims for Patients

- Within three months, each person with advanced dementia will have relief from pain and discomfort, as measured by the PAIN-AD scale (see Chapter 4 for details on pain relief).
- Within three months, patients' crying out will be reduced by 75% by addressing underlying causes of this behavior and treating them.
- All people who can bear weight now will be able to bear weight six months from now (except for those who are admitted to hospice care).
- Within three months, 85% of patients with advanced dementia can be assisted with Activities of Daily Living (ADLs) without exhibiting resistive behaviors.
- Within three months, all people with dementia will receive complementary therapies, such as music, massage, and "positive interactions," as indicated in their care plans, for at least one hour every day.
- By next year, 90% of the records for deceased advanced dementia patients will show documentation that each patient's (and that patient's family's) end-of-life treatment decisions

were respected (e.g., concerning hospitalizations, antibiotics, feeding tubes, CPR, and so forth).

- For next year's record of family evaluation of care, 90% of family members will agree or strongly agree with the following statements: "I felt that my family member with advanced dementia was respected during the last phase of life"; "My family member did not suffer during the last phase of life."

- On the staff survey next year, 100% of staff will report that they had cared fully and appropriately for patients with advanced dementia.

Aims for Caregivers

On the next bereavement survey:

- Ninety percent of families will report that they received the help and support that they needed following a loved one's death.

On next year's family evaluation of care:

- Seventy-five percent of families will report that they had the time to take care of things they needed to do during their loved one's last phase of life.

- Eighty-five percent of families will respond that there were no surprises in the course of the disease or with the professional care given.

- One hundred percent of family members will say that they knew where to turn for answers to their questions.

- One hundred percent of family members will say that they felt supported by staff during their loved one's last phase of life.

- One hundred percent of families will say that they participated in the care of their loved one as they wished.

- Ninety percent of those family members using respite care will report that respite caregivers provided appropriate care and that they felt comfortable leaving the patient with the respite companion.

As you develop your aim, remember that some people with advanced dementia do not appear to be experiencing pain, even when they have been assessed with a dementia-specific scale. It can be difficult to know when the person is suffering from physical distress, much less knowing when the person is nearing death. Sometimes we think, "How much longer can the patient live like this?" Monitoring and assessing pain, discomfort, pressure ulcers, intake and output, and activity levels can help you and the patient's family to recognize how the disease is progressing.

The criteria available to predict death for people with dementia within the next six months are not helpful. Families need to understand that they are living with an unpredictable illness—but they also need to be confident that they are doing so with reliable care and support. With this awareness, they can prepare for the end and think about the inevitable treatment decisions.

Families need help understanding that *not* pursuing aggressive medical treatments (i.e., feeding tubes, antibiotics near the end of life, unnecessary hospitalizations, CPR) does not equal not caring. Most research studies show that these interventions do not improve the quality or length of life. Family members have to consider palliative care and to weigh which measures are likely to be helpful. Often, family members will need time to discuss and agree on a treatment plan because the patient is unable to make healthcare decisions.

No matter which aim you choose, you are likely to see improvement in other areas, too. For instance, if you work on improving patients' exposure to human touch and engagement, you are likely to see fewer family complaints and improved staff morale, as well as a decrease in the frequency of patients' disruptive behavior. You may want to measure outcomes in these areas.

While you will be measuring process goals (e.g., how well are we doing in implementing the change?), always keep in mind that finding some way to measure the outcome, that is, the benefit to the patient and the family, is the most important goal.

CHOOSING A TEAM

TEAM SUNSHINE

Team members agreed that while they knew their participants fairly well and had a feel for how to set up a project on human touch and engagement, they did not know much about QI. The director knew someone at the Alzheimer's Association who had experience in QI and in advanced dementia and asked her to help. They also asked a doctor who had many patients at the center if they could call her occasionally for her perspective. Finally, they invited an activist family member to join them. The team had an aim, and it had a structure: a day-to-day leader, a data collection and analysis person, staff directly involved in participant care, and a QI expert with contacts at other facilities. The family member agreed to keep in touch with other family members about the project's progress.

As you build your QI team, think strategically, and involve people who share your enthusiasm for the work—and for the patients. Include people who are directly involved in the process itself and whose work will be affected by the outcomes. Involve senior leaders, especially those who can approve and support your project and bring resources to bear.

When you embark on a QI project, take time to discuss teamwork. Everyone should agree on the aim and should know that it cannot be accomplished by one person alone. If you are the team leader, you will need to keep the QI project on target; sometimes, teams can be sidetracked and lose focus.

MEASURING SUCCESS

TEAM SUNSHINE

The QI expert suggested changes, but the team was reluctant to start until they had a clear sense of how to measure their work. Instead, they decided to make a simple chart that showed how each participant was spending time between meals. The chart listed each participant's name in columns and had rows labeled with participant activities, both positive and negative. The team agreed on what should be listed as negative behaviors, including sleeping, crying out, staring off into space, sitting alone, and so forth. Positive behaviors by patients included tapping their feet or nodding their heads to the music, looking at the caregiver, receiving a hand massage or manicure, receiving a foot mas-

Table 10.1 Team Sunshine Activity Log

Time of Observation	10:00 A.M.		
Name	Positive activity/comment	Negative activity/comment	ADL/comment
Mary	xx/hair brushed		
Joe	xx/looked at photos		
Jane		xx/asleep in chair	
Joseph	xx/walk to activity		
Michael		xx/asleep in chair	
Amy			x/lift to stand
Claudia		xx/grimacing, crying	

sage, getting their hair brushed, or having makeup applied. The chart also had a column for patients receiving ADL care.

Knowing that they did not need or want to collect baseline data forever in order to prove their point, the three hands-on staff members decided to track three participants every half hour between lunch and dinner for four days. They then gave the data to the director for analysis. She found that participants were exhibiting the sleeping, crying, staring, fidgeting, and solitary behaviors 75% of the time and were only involved in positive activities 25% of the time. Clearly, the team had much improvement to do in order to reach its 90% positive rate.

The team decided to measure the percentage of positive activities that Sunshine Club members were engaged in during nonmeal and toileting times (their sample) because they knew they could not keep up with observing and charting every half hour, every day, for the next six months. Since they already used a "day sheet" to check participants hourly, they added a column to check observations of positive activity. The team checked two day sheets per week, varying the days reviewed. Simple instructions were printed on the back of the day sheet. The measurement tool was in place, and the team was poised to begin implementing activity changes.

Before introducing new paperwork, look at the data your organization now collects to see if you can adapt it for your use. People are much more likely to maintain changes and continue measurements when it is simpler to perform the new behavior than it is to do things the old way.

If your organization does a yearly satisfaction survey, see if you can add one or two outcome measures that will reflect your progress over time. If your families and staff fill out a bereavement satisfaction survey, include outcome measures on it. For some changes—for example, for 100% of patients to have advanced care directives—it may take little time to collect outcome data that show progress. Other changes, like family reflections on patient suffering, bereavement, and making the right treatment decisions, may be collected in routine family surveys.

Promising tools are available to measure changes in comfort for people with advanced dementia since they cannot report their own symptoms. One of these is the PAIN-AD (see Chapter 4); another, the Non-Communicative Patient's Pain Assessment Instrument (NOPPAIN), is geared for use by nursing assistants when giving physical care. Family members can easily use it to report information to the healthcare provider. Other tools used to measure comfort may be less useful, especially if they rely on patient reports. Often, professional and family caregivers must rely on observations and changes from previous behaviors to track changes in behaviors or symptoms. Even these informal observations can be data sources.

While you will be measuring process goals (how well you are doing in implementing the change), always keep in mind that finding some way to measure outcomes—the benefit to the patient and the family—is the most important goal.

The following lists recommend measures for comfort, appropriate care, and caregiver aims:

Comfort Aims

- Daily (or more frequently, if needed) pain and comfort assessments.
- Medication records that reflect the effects of pain medications and assessment of these records within two hours of administration.
- Care plans that contain appropriate activities and interactions based on the person's history, including music, massage, religious readings/practices, and so forth.
- Patients who can maintain a standing position for five

minutes (excluding those who have been transferred to hospice care).

- Patients who do not exhibit untoward behaviors during the day or evening shifts.
- People who eat half of their meals with caregivers seated beside them, not standing over them, for assistance.
- Patients who maintain a desirable weight until they are referred for hospice services.
- People who do not develop pressure ulcers.

Appropriate Care Aims

- People die outside the hospital who had expressed (or whose family expressed) a desire not to be hospitalized.
- People who developed infections were treated according to family decisions.
- Feeding tubes not being inserted (except for those whose decision-makers understood the options well and still chose tube feeding).
- Family members expressing belief that their loved one did not suffer near the end.
- Family members who agree that the patient was treated with respect in the last phase of life.
- Patients with dementia had a family member, caregiver, or volunteer in attendance around the clock for the last week of life.

Caregiver Aims

- Family members who report that they were able to continue daily activities beyond caregiving.
- Families who report on bereavement surveys that they received the comfort, education, and respite that they needed during the last phase of their family member's life.
- Family caregivers who agree that they participated in their family member's care as they had wished.

- Families who report that there were no surprises for them in their loved one's last phase of life.
- Staff who felt that they were able to do all that they could to help people in advanced stages of dementia.
- Staff caregivers who feel supported by the organization as they work through their own grief when patients in their care have died.

CHANGES TO TRY

TEAM SUNSHINE

The group tried several successive changes, each building on the last. The first was to instruct staff members in how to follow the revised day sheet to track project data (Change 1). It took almost two weeks before everyone was filling out the day sheet consistently and was clear about what to classify as a "positive activity" and how to mark it accordingly. This move, however, resulted in no change in the percentage of people engaged in positive activities.

Next, the team implemented hand massage, manicures, makeup application, and other grooming activities after breakfast (Change 2). The staff, who were used to assisting with ADLs, seemed to enjoy this activity, too, and chatted with participants and one another. A beauty supply store donated lotion samples, and some participants could even continue rubbing their own hands together after the hand lotion was applied. Pulling hair back and applying light lipstick to the women who were used to wearing cosmetics encouraged other staff and visitors to comment to the patients, "How nice you look today."

After two weeks, participation in positive activities had jumped to 40%. The team was delighted to find that participants became more responsive, often holding their hands out for lotion and smiling more at their caregivers. Indeed, it actually felt like a Sunshine Club!

Your aim statement will drive the nature of the changes that you try. Remember, try one change at a time, and determine whether it is an improvement, before spreading it to more patients or embarking on the next one. Depending on your patients' needs and your resources, you may be able to try the breadth of changes, like those for the Sunshine Club, or you may want to narrow your scope. Here is a list of changes that other teams have tried:

- Build in steps in each CNA's career ladder which acknowledge care given beyond ADLs, such as training provided to other staff and the use of symptom-monitoring scales.
- Invite CNAs to care planning meetings.
- Include implementing activity programs/services in staff evaluations.
- Share findings of family surveys with hands-on staff.
- Add staffing hours to help out with ADLs and activity programs by recruiting students, volunteers, and interns.
- Provide a monthly activity calendar that shows group activities for both higher and lower functioning participants.
- Modify your environment to enhance the abilities of participants to become engaged. For instance, decrease overhead loudspeakers, decrease staff talking to one another when they are more than three feet apart, and seat participants in conversational settings rather than lined up against a wall.
- Implement dementia-specific communication strategies.
- Ask staff to tell you at least three things about each participant's life before the patient was afflicted with dementia.

TELLING YOUR STORY: TIME SERIES GRAPH

The Sunshine Club measured and tracked positive behaviors, which it graphed in a time series chart. Such graphs are effective ways to communicate which changes were tested and whether progress was made.

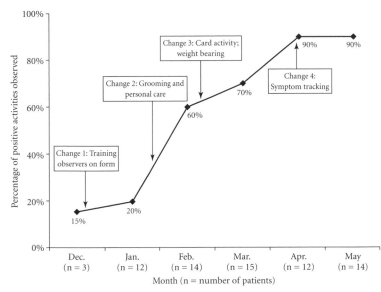

FIGURE 10.1 Improvement in positive behaviors. In five months, the Sunshine Club participants will have human contact and engagement in positive activities when observed, at least 90% of the monitoring times.

TEAM SUNSHINE

One change was introduced as much to help the team as to help the participants. The staff wondered how family caregivers managed participants at home since it might take two of the staff just to raise someone out of the chair and assist the person to stand during transfer. Families had donated old greeting cards and magazines to the program, so staff put a selection of these on the table, seated the participants around the table, and began looking through the items with participants. Eventually, patients began picking up items that interested them, examining them, and then picking up another. One staff person sat between two people who were less able to look at the items on their own and carried on something of a monologue for the participants, picking

*up things that she thought might be of interest to them. In the mean-
time, two staffers moved about the room and helped everyone at the
table to a standing position and supported or guarded them while they
stood for up to five minutes at a time. Then they helped the person sit
down and moved on to the next person. Eventually, the staff found that
this simple activity helped people bear their own weight during transfers for quite a while. Mostly, this little exercise kept participants able
to help in transfers until they weakened and were admitted to hospice
services. Staff and family alike were amazed that this simple intervention could make such a difference!*

Give Them Something to Talk About

Team Sunshine

*Based on the team's success, the director amended the yearly budget to
purchase supplies for the Sunshine Club and began asking families to
donate supplies (e.g., nail polish, lotion, magazines). Knowing that the
director supported its work was great news for the Sunshine Club, and
the director also agreed to work with the team to train volunteers each
month so as to free up the direct care staff and to have more people
who could engage with participants.*

*The Alzheimer's Association representative called a nurse friend and
asked her to help the staff learn more about symptom management,
thinking that some patient behaviors reflected pain and discomfort. The
nurse spent an afternoon training staff to use the NOPPAIN tool. With
family permission, physicians were contacted when participants evi-
denced pain symptoms. Sometimes, relief was as simple as moving the
person from a wheelchair to a straight-backed chair for a while each
day.*

After the fourth month, the team reached its goal of 90%. Delighted with their success and the results that they saw with participants, the team decided that they could not stop there, and they eventually went on to try QI projects to address family caregiver issues and treatment decision issues.

So many little things add up to good palliative care for people with advanced dementia. Keeping both the person with dementia and the caregiver educated and supported during the early phases of the illness matters, and so does recognizing that caring for people with dementia requires more that just good hygiene and feeding.

Tools and Resources

- Alzheimer's Association Campaign for Quality Residential Care: Dementia Care Practice Recommendations for Assisted Living Residences and Nursing Homes (2005) http://www.alz.org
- Caring for a Loved One with Advanced Dementia: A Caregiver's Manual http://www.hom.org
- NOPPAIN (Non-Communicative Patient's Pain Assessment Instrument) by Snow, A. L., O'Malley, K., Kunic, M., Cody, M., Beck, C., & Ashton, C. http://www.sdfmc.org/ClassLibrary/Page/Information/ DataInstances/81/Files/339/noppainform_1.pdf
- Pain Assessment in Advanced Dementia (PAINAD) http://mqa.dhs.state.tx.us/QMWeb/Pain/PAINAD.htm

11

IMPROVING INTENSIVE CARE UNITS

IN THIS CHAPTER

- Offering palliative care in the intensive care unit (ICU)
- Identifying patients likely to die in ICU and unmet needs
- Using time-limited trials for patients who do not forgo treatment
- Managing ventilator weaning and withdrawal
- Supporting family and other caregivers

The intensive care unit traditionally focuses on medical interventions to save and prolong life, and most patients and families cling to the hope of recovery and cure. But the fact is that people die in the ICU, often because of an exacerbation of a chronic illness. For those patients for whom one more rescue turns out not to be possible, the ICU can offer comfort and solace through palliative care services, including symptom management and family support. For some ICU patients, of course, there is little warning that death is imminent. But for others, especially those with chronic disease, when the odds for death seem very likely, physicians and nurses can take steps to improve the level of symptom management, to support and aid families, and to assist in ventilator withdrawal.

This chapter describes steps that you can try in the ICU in order to improve care for dying patients and their families. It provides examples of successful programs developed by other quality improvement (QI) teams. By following the basic QI process described in Chapter 2, you too can develop a successful project. Team Dudley is a composite based on many groups that have successfully improved their care for end-of life-patients in the ICU.

TEAM DUDLEY

The mission statement for University Hospital's Palliative Care Program perfectly captures Team Dudley's desire to care for the dying: The team is dedicated to alleviating suffering, providing high-quality pain and symptom management, and supporting patient-centered care for those with serious illness and their families through comprehensive educational programs, and innovative research in palliative care. Putting this into practice in the ICU has been challenging for the hospital. Its medical director wants to initiate and evaluate a systematic, proactive palliative care consultation for ICU patients who are at high risk of dying. What might Team Dudley do?

IDENTIFYING THE PROBLEM AND SETTING AN AIM

As many as three quarters of ICU patients with cancer experience pain, anxiety, sleep disorders, or unsatisfied hunger or thirst. Chances are that patients feel like this in your ICU. Patients nearing the end of life benefit from palliative care that focuses on appropriate treatment, comfort measures, and family support. Before deciding to launch palliative care consults, first look closely at your ICU patients to determine which symptoms most trouble them and what can be done to improve their care. Is unrelieved pain really ignored, or is it that it takes too long to get medication? Are families unprepared for the process of ventilator withdrawal? Is there a protocol for explaining the situation to families, for letting them know what is happening and why?

Based on the needs that your team members identify, develop an aim statement.

TEAM DUDLEY

First, Team Dudley met to discuss what each member observed, what existing data showed, and where improvement was needed. The team was surprised to find that most of its palliative care consult requests in the ICU were referred more than 15 days after admission. As a result, the team set the three following aims:

Aim 1: On each patient's first day in the medical intensive care unit (MICU), identify those patients at high risk of in-hospital death, and refer at least 80% of them to palliative care before death or discharge. Achieve this aim within 90 days.

Aim 2: For these patients, decrease the number of days between MICU admission and palliative care consult to two, down from the current 15.

Aim 3: Increase the use of time-limited trials to 100% of patients receiving palliative care consults who do not forgo ventilators, artificial feeding, and other potentially life-prolonging treatment.

Take a look at these three statements again. Do any include all four components of an effective aim statement? The first aim does.

What will improve: *Identification and referral of high-risk patients to palliative care.*

By when: *Within 90 days.*

By how much: *Up to 80% of the target population.*

For whom: *ICU patients at high risk of death during this period of hospitalization.*

CHOOSING A TEAM

TEAM DUDLEY

With Team Dudley's aims set, the lead ICU physician and nurse began to think about colleagues whose involvement seemed important. Eventually, the team grew to include another ICU physician, two critical care nurses, a palliative care consultant, and a data manager. By detailing its aim and what it hoped to accomplish, the team convinced senior hospital leadership to support their work. With support from the director of palliative care, the chief quality officer, and chief medical officer, the team had access to resources and staff that could help to make sure that the project would work.

By now, you may be curious as to why the team chose to call themselves "Team Dudley." The team borrowed the name from the cartoon character Dudley Do-Right, of course, because they intended to learn how to do it right.

A good idea might provide the basis for a good QI project, but a great project only happens with the involvement of key players, both on the QI team and in the organization's management. Deciding which of your colleagues to involve is one important step, and recognizing whether you are missing key players is another. Including stakeholders from each area is the key to good team support. You might also want to add a patient advocate or ethicist, someone who can speak to the needs and interests of patients and families. Remember to try including the following staff:

- An administrative person who will champion your cause.
- Someone who knows QI methods.
- Someone who knows a lot about critical care practice, such as a critical care nurse.

MEASURING SUCCESS

Whatever your aim, the rapid-cycle improvement process relies on three basic measure types: outcome, process, and adverse effects (see Chapter 2). Your team needs to decide which data to collect, who will collect it and when, and whether and how to sample.

TEAM DUDLEY

Once the team had its aim and membership in place, the group worked out the specifics of how to measure whether its efforts were making a difference. Based on its aim statements, the team came up with the following outcome measures.

Outcome measure 1: *For patients referred to palliative care, have a nurse provide bedside assessment of the patient's comfort level by the end of the next eight-hour shift.*

Outcome measure 2: *The length of the patient's stay in the ICU.*

Adverse-effect measure: *Family complaints about discussions of the prognosis and care options.*

Although these were perfectly good measures, it only took a few weeks for the team to see that they had listed three aims that dealt only with the processes of care, and that they were using measures that focused upon outcomes. Thus, their aims and measures did not match closely. Sometimes the process and outcome are so closely aligned that not much turns on the distinction. But that was not the case here. The team went back to work on getting their aims and measures to match. They realized that what they had labeled as aims were really changes and that what really mattered was what was latent in the measures. On this basis, they changed their aims.

Aim 1: *Within six months, at least 80% of patients who have 70% or higher risk of dying during this hospitalization (by the Acute Physiology and Chronic Health Evaluation [APACHE] scoring*

*system) will be assessed as being comfortable by their nurse by
the end of the second day's daytime shift.*

Aim 2: *For these high-risk patients, the average length of stay in the
ICU will decline by one half.*

Then, the matching measures are obvious.

Measure 1: *The comfort rating on second hospital day among ICU
patients likely to die.*

Measure 2: *The length of stay in the ICU among ICU patients likely
to die.*

There are many outcomes to measure progress in your ICU QI program. The following list might inspire you to think about what is important in your environment:

- palliative care symptom scores;
- collaboration and satisfaction with decision-making (among families and ICU staff);
- congruency of patient treatment and goals;
- loved ones' perception of patient suffering;
- ICU discharge: mortality and transfer rates;
- ICU and hospital lengths of stay;
- family follow-up surveys for those that had loved ones die in the ICU.

TELLING YOUR STORY: TIME SERIES GRAPH

Most QI teams find it effective to track their work on a simple time series chart.

TEAM DUDLEY

Team Dudley came up with a chart that shows the proportion of eligible patients who had a palliative care consult (see Figure 11.1). They also graphed the number of days between the ICU admission and the consult. From a baseline of 15 days, the team eventually got this number down to five days in the first quarter and two days in the second quarter. The hospital's information technology (IT) group provided these data. Figure 11.2 shows the time series graph for the patients' length of ICU stay.

Figure 11.2 shows the major interventions and setbacks, and there is clearly a strong trend toward shorter lengths of stay. However, the QI team receiving these data also picked up a very important additional trend. The number of patients with very poor prognosis who were in the ICU was declining. The number of high-risk patients went from 32 in June to 20 in November. A little investigation confirmed their

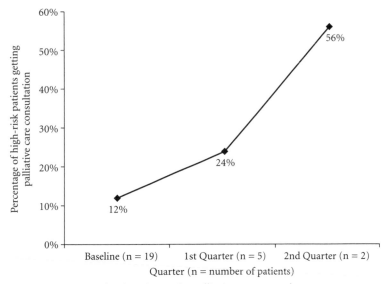

FIGURE 11.1 Monitoring change in palliative care consult rate.

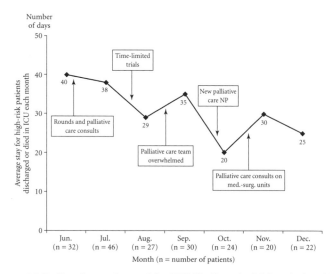

FIGURE 11.2 Aim: For patients with >70% likelihood of dying during this hospitalization; length of stay in ICU

hunch that the clinicians on the medical unit, backed by consultations with the palliative care team there, had started making better advance care plans (ACPs) with desperately ill patients and their families, and fewer were being transferred to ICU. Since the decisions reflected good care, and since the ICU was still filled with patients with better prognoses, this was a good result from all perspectives.

IDENTIFYING AND TESTING CHANGES

TEAM DUDLEY

In order to reach its aims, Team Dudley had to come up with changes that it wanted to test. It first decided to use a screening tool to identify patients who were likely to benefit from a palliative care consult. Criteria included the following:

- *Admission to the ICU following a hospital stay of at least 10 days.*
- *Age greater than 80, with two or more eventually fatal conditions.*
- *Diagnosis of an incurable malignancy.*
- *Survival following a cardiac arrest.*
- *Intracerebral hemorrhaging requiring mechanical ventilation.*

A liaison who was a full-time palliative care nurse practitioner began to make rounds with the MICU staff and to implement the screening tool. Within days, the nurse practitioner realized that the ICU calculated APACHE scores on every patient every day, so the data on the statistical likelihood of a patient dying during this hospitalization was available and much easier to use. That observation shaped the recasting of the aim described above. The team decided to encourage the use of time-limited trials using a brief script. The palliative care nurse introduced the idea to family decision-makers that a patient might be on tube-feedings or another treatment for one week (or another specified time), and then if no progress was made, the treatment would end. The team did not try each change at the same time but rather phased in changes over the course of several weeks.

Once the basic process and aim have been set, your team will need to develop changes to test. Remember that each change will not necessarily lead to the improvement that you envision. When you are stuck, or when the change just does not seem to be working, then stop. Think about what you need to vary, or reconsider to make the change more effective—and thus retool your project. This process teaches you a great deal about how your system really works. Successful ICU changes that have been tried by other QI teams include:

- standardizing protocols;
- regular ethics rounds in the ICU;

- time-limited trials for interventions such as ventilators, artificial nutrition, and hydration;
- early identification of patients who need palliative care;
- pain as a "Fifth Vital Sign" for all patients;
- direct family support, including providing them with telephones and pagers, showers, and a place to rest;
- competent management of ventilator withdrawal.

Time-Limited Trials

It is often hard for patients or their family members to choose between various treatment options, especially when they do not know which treatment will provide the comfort and quality of life that they are looking for. They think that once they start the treatment, they will not be able to stop it. In situations like these, when there is any doubt about whether a treatment will improve a patient's comfort or quality of life, a time-limited trial is very useful. *Time-limited trial* means trying a treatment for a reasonable period of time to see if the patient benefits. The key is to define the time limit and the expected benefits before starting the treatment. That way, everyone will know when the situation will be reassessed and what benefits should be present to consider the treatment useful.

More information related to ventilator withdrawal techniques and how to prepare for it is given below. A protocol for medications used in ventilator withdrawal and a checklist of important considerations can be found in *Improving Care at the End of Life: A Sourcebook for Clinicians and Managers* (http://www.mywhatever.com/cifwriter/content/66/4205.html).

Ventilator Withdrawal Techniques

1. Rapid weaning:
   - affords the most control;
   - when used for awake and aware patients, negotiate a plan and follow it;

- when used for cognitively impaired patients, be sure that treatment prevents suffering.
- a novice clinician conducting withdrawal must have an experienced clinician at hand.

2. Immediate transfer to a t-bar/tracheotomy collar:
   - patients who are comatose without cognition (e.g., global cerebral ischemia).
   - patients may breathe for a while, and the intubation allows easy suctioning.

3. Extubation:
   - for patients who are brain dead when testing shows that there will be no effort to breathe.
   - declare death before extubation.

How to Prepare for Ventilator Withdrawal

1. Prior to Withdrawal:
   - discontinue all medications, tests, and treatment not directed toward comfort care;
   - remove unnecessary lines and tubes;
   - maintain one IV access site for administration of analgesia and sedation;
   - determine noninvasive monitoring needs;
   - discontinue unnecessary alarm systems, including internal defibrillator devices or pacemakers;
   - assemble equipment and medication necessary for comfort and pain control;
   - provide a quiet atmosphere and unlimited visiting hours for families;
   - ensure that caregivers who are uncomfortable with the process can withdraw from the case;
   - involve the chaplain or the family's religious supports, as appropriate;

- support family members who are staying with their loved one.

2. Withdrawal:
   - the attending physician and chaplain are usually present;
   - raise the head of the bed, if possible;
   - clear the airways of secretions if necessary, for both patient comfort and to reduce the anxiety of the family;
   - administer and maintain appropriate levels of sedation/ analgesia for signs of dyspnea and distress;
   - reduce ventilator settings so as to provide minimal support, or remove the patient from the ventilator;
   - extubate the patient and, if indicated, place the patient on oxygen as a comfort measure.

COMMON BARRIERS TO GOOD MANAGEMENT

TEAM DUDLEY

Once the team had established the palliative care consultation program, the demand for its services grew rapidly. The team struggled to meet the growing demand and eventually persuaded the administrators to hire a new nurse practitioner. Even after success in their project, they continued to have to make the case for additional resources to expand the service to other units.

All improvement efforts encounter barriers. Anticipating and preparing for them will allow your team to overcome problems while staying focused on your aim. Table 11.1 shows barriers to expect in the ICU and how you can overcome them.

Table 11.1 Barriers and Solutions

Barriers to Providing Good Care in ICU	What You Can Do
<ul><li>Patients and family members believe that the ICU can offer remarkable control over recovery and death.</li><li>Patients may rely on family members for decision-making, and families do not always agree on a decision.</li><li>Families hear differing viewpoints, primarily from a variety of physician specialists, which can lead to confusion and frustration.</li><li>Healthcare team members may not agree on diagnosis or treatment options, or they may have personal issues about death and dying that limit their ability to communicate with patients and their families.</li><li>Providers are reluctant to speak to families about death and involve them in decision-making.</li><li>Palliative care is introduced very late in the process when all other interventions have failed.</li></ul>	<ul><li>Provide accurate information about prognosis and options.</li><li>Help family (and patients, if possible) make plans for dying, just in case things do not go well (see Chapter 8).</li><li>Hold meetings/conferences with family members to talk about all aspects of care.</li><li>Focus on discussing patients' likely preferences. Bring any written documentation from the patient, such as an advance directive or proxy form.</li><li>Involve the treating and primary physician early on in discussions.</li><li>Regularly offer support to physicians in facilitating these discussions.</li><li>Channel information to each family through one physician or nurse.</li><li>Hold regular team meetings to discuss each patient and agree on the treatment protocol.</li><li>Provide training and support to providers to deal with these issues.</li><li>Offer in-service training programs based on palliative care education series offered by medical and nursing organizations.</li><li>Identify patients early by proactively screening them. Have the screening criteria known to everyone.</li><li>Include palliative care consultants to regular ICU team.</li></ul>

Give Them Something to Talk About

Team Dudley

Once Team Dudley had met its goal and the project had ended, the team wanted to be sure that its progress did not slip. The team convinced the hospital administrators to hire a full-time person to identify ICU patients for palliative care and to work with them and their families. The process was set up in such a way that these consultations take place routinely. The team continues to track cost data that compare patients at high risk of dying who did not receive a consult (standard care) with those who did. This information has convinced administrators that the ideas and techniques benefit patients in a cost-effective manner. Consideration is being given to expanding palliative care to other ICUs in the hospital.

12

BUILDING A PALLIATIVE CARE PROGRAM

IN THIS CHAPTER

- Decisions about whether to launch a palliative care program
- Ways to manage palliative care program development
- Evaluating a palliative care program

Encouraged by their success in establishing components of good palliative care, some quality improvement (QI) teams decide to establish palliative care programs. These ambitious teams are to be encouraged and applauded, but they are also to be cautioned: setting up an entirely new hospital-based program is *not* a QI project. It requires a different approach, one that entails mostly program structure and function, including how the endeavor will be staffed and funded. With the rapid-cycle QI method, we advocate an approach that thrives on a quick study, repeated tests of new ideas (with the option to discard those that do not work), and a gradual spread to a larger population. Creating a new program, on the other hand, demands that you review a lot of data, talk to many people, consider several options, and then gamble on one substantial change.

From a QI perspective, palliative care programs are:

- a change worth trying—probably not the first and certainly not the last;

- a locus of responsibility for ongoing improvements, a natural home for repeated QI;
- a major structure for sustaining improvements.

For those looking to start a palliative care program, we offer this chapter. Here, we focus on the work that needs to be done before starting a program and on issues to consider when laying the groundwork.

Models for palliative care programs take a few basic forms: scattered inpatient beds, dedicated hospital units, consult services, or outpatient clinics. Your choice will depend on your patient demographics, what patients and families need, what clinicians want, your resources, and the willingness of hospital leadership to change.

This section discusses the clinical and organizational structure that undergirds a good palliative care program. Keep in mind that setting up a program is not really a suitable goal for a rapid-cycle QI project; it goes far beyond the scope of such an effort. If you want to set up a program, that is great. But remember, once you have it going, you should still pursue patient-centered QI goals, for example: a reduction in pain scores, fewer unexpected hospitalizations of frail elders, more prompt referrals to hospice, and so forth.

For more detailed information, we recommend programs and resources sponsored by the Center to Advance Palliative Care (CAPC) at http://www.capc.org.

What Is Palliative Care?

The World Health Organization defines palliative care as "the active total care of patients whose disease is not responsive to curative treatment . . . [when] control of pain, of other symptoms, and of psychological, social and spiritual problems is paramount" (WHO, 1990). Palliative care is often described as a way to meet the physical, mental, and spiritual needs of chronically ill and dying patients. Clinicians may tend to associate palliative care with oncology and believe that it is what is done when aggressive, curative treatment no longer works. Many clinicians think there is a demarcation line between when cure-oriented care ends and palliative care begins; others believe the transition is far more gradual and less clear-cut. Clinicians may believe that to receive palliative care, patients must forgo other treatments, such as radiation or chemotherapy, when in fact palliative care may be appropriate at any time, including during disease modifying treatment.

What Is a Palliative Care Program?

Palliative care programs share several goals: to provide treatment for pain management and other symptom control; to give patients and families information needed to make the best treatment decisions possible, including whether to forgo treatment; to offer emotional support and practical assistance to patients and families; and to organize coordinated, comprehensive care, in the hospital and at home.

Are Palliative Care and Hospice the Same Thing?

Although palliative care and hospice share common goals for patient comfort, they are different in several essential ways. Table 12.1 describes the differences between palliative care, hospice, geriatrics, and case management.

Why Are Palliative Care Programs Important?

Palliative care programs are important because they offer a way to provide comprehensive services, starting with care planning and symptom management, for people living with life-limiting illnesses. Such programs

Table 12.1 Palliative Care versus Related Services

	Palliative Care	Geriatrics	Hospice Care	Case Management
Patients Served	Patients of any age, suffering with life-threatening illnesses.	Elderly and frail patients.	Dying patients of any age.	All patients with complex care needs.
Services Provided	Throughout illness, and simultaneous with other treatment: comprehensive, coordinated pain and symptom control, care of psychological and spiritual needs, family support and assistance in making transitions between care settings.	Prevention, rehabilitation, disease management, functional assessment, and recovery specific to older adults.	At the end of life or when curative treatments are not desired or not effective: comprehensive, coordinated pain and symptom control, care of psychological and spiritual needs, family support, and assistance in making transitions between care settings. Bereavement care for survivors.	Assists to develop treatment plans guided by benchmarks, pathways, and standards.

Key Differences			
Program open to all seriously ill patients, not just those with six-month prognosis. Patients do not have to forgo curative care. Palliative care team coordinates care from a variety of healthcare providers, including specialists and primary-care physicians.	Focus on prevention, chronic disease management, functional assessment, recovery, and rehabilitation among older adults.	Six-month prognosis required by Medicare and other payers. Coverage includes outpatient medications and supplies. Efforts to cure or prolong life are not covered by Medicare hospice benefit.	Assists to coordinate care and facilitate transitions between settings. Independent medical judgment not intrinsic.

209

are a way to coordinate services for critically ill and dying patients across the disparate units of hospitals and sometimes across the patchwork of disparate programs outside of hospitals.

For patients, palliative care programs are a reliable approach of coordinated and comprehensive care to the all-too-confusing world of healthcare. Palliative care itself offers ongoing comfort and treatment, as well as support in making the difficult decisions near the end of life.

For institutions, palliative care programs are an effective and efficient way to care for the growing number of patients who have severe, chronic conditions requiring repeated hospitalizations. Without such a program, hospitals will struggle financially as they provide increasingly expensive, high-intensity care for more patients who have more frequent hospitalizations. In addition, a palliative care program can help hospitals meet Joint Commission on Accreditation of Healthcare Organizations (JCAHO) standards for pain management.

Finally, clinicians find that palliative care programs offer a way to improve bedside management of pain and other distress through consults with palliative care experts. This approach fosters patient and family satisfaction while saving physicians time, helping them to manage the more time-intensive aspects of care, such as communicating with patients and families, coordinating care across settings, and managing difficult symptoms.

What Are the Arguments for Palliative Care?

Diane Meier, MD, founder and director of the Center to Advance Palliative Care, based at the Mount Sinai School of Medicine in New York City, gives five basic arguments for offering a palliative care service:

1. To enhance clinical quality by meeting the need for better quality of care for people with serious, complex, and life-limiting illnesses.

2. To ensure meeting patient and family preferences for better symptom relief, such as more contact with healthcare professionals, improved emotional support, and guidance for the challenges of caregiving.

3. To respond to demographics; with predictions of 10 million people in the United States ages 85 and older by the year 2030, healthcare must change to meet the needs of patients with multiple chronic conditions.

4. To increase educational opportunities for physicians, many of whom have little or no formal training in end-of-life care.

5. To reduce costs. The current combination of financing healthcare, burgeoning costs, and increasing technology, combined with an aging (and, eventually, ailing) population, will spell financial disaster. Palliative care programs decrease the length of stay and reduce costs while providing good, compassionate care that is in line with patient preferences.

What kinds of care will be classified as palliative care, and which patients will be the primary "customers"? Will services be offered on an institution-wide level or limited to a dedicated unit? Do you want to start with a consult service? Who will you include on the palliative care team—physicians, nurses, social workers, nutritionists, clergy, volunteers?

Is There a Process for Starting a Program?

The first step is to assess needs. Examine patient and family needs, especially diagnoses and treatment patterns. A record review is the most effective method for this: look at pain and other symptom scores, reasons for readmissions and lengths of stay, treatment, advance care plans, and consults.

What types of care are you providing now for patients with chronic, life-limiting illnesses? Are pain and other symptoms assessed and treated? What kind of quality of life do your patients have? (Are they in and out of the hospital, mobile, isolated?) What are their care preferences? Are most of your patients seeking cures, despite evidence that they are nearing the end of life? Are patients and families satisfied with your current services?

Consider the institution's mission and vision, and think about how a palliative care program might fit within these. The size and scope of palliative care services can vary dramatically, and they often depend on the space available for dedicated palliative care beds. What is staffing like? How is your staff's morale? What is your institution's bed occupancy? Can the current staff take on a new project, or will you need more resources?

Palliative care programs rely on the interaction of many organizations and functions: hospital consults; ambulatory outpatient, inpatient, and residential hospice; home healthcare; home hospice; nursing homes. Orchestrating their interaction can be a complex task, both from an institutional vantage and from the patient's perspective. A palliative care service can be the ideal vehicle to accomplish this.

What Kinds of Programs Work Best?

There are four basic models for palliative care programs: inpatient beds scattered throughout a hospital; dedicated inpatient units; consult services; and outpatient clinics. According to palliative care expert Charles von Gunten, MD, there are four issues in deciding which model will work best: (1) What does the institution need? (2) What is possible? (3) What is easy (and can be done)? (4) Where is the support coming from? If dedicated beds are not available, a consult service is the best option. If there are empty beds or units, then dedicated beds or an inpatient unit might work. In general, smaller hospitals tend to start with consult services, while larger ones, especially teaching hospitals, can support a dedicated unit and service. What are the strengths and weakness of each type of program?

Choosing a Program Model

As you decide which program is right for your patients, consider the following questions:

- What problem(s) will a palliative care program address?
- Will a palliative care unit or consultation service provide part of the solution?
- What other elements are needed to solve the problem(s) identified?
- Can the program be sustained financially? How will it be funded?
- How will providers bill for care?
- What effect will the unit or service have on overall costs?
- Which staff members are available? Will new staff be hired or even be necessary? How much and what kind of training will be needed?
- How will the group measure its progress?

Strategies for gathering this kind of information can include:

- retrospective chart reviews, both qualitative and quantitative;
- inpatient questionnaires and interviews;
- family questionnaires and interviews, by phone or in focus groups;
- focus groups with physicians, nurses, medical students, and others;
- roundtable discussions with house staff;

- management information system (MIS) data on hospital deaths;
- monitoring and assessment of a select group of current end-of-life patients.

How Are Programs Staffed?

The National Consensus Project on Clinical Practice Guidelines for Quality Palliative Care reports that specialty-level palliative care is best delivered through an interdisciplinary team consisting of appropriately trained and credentialed physicians, nurses, and social workers. Additional support and contributions can come from chaplains, rehabilitation experts, psychiatrists, and other professionals. Ultimately, the needs and capacities of the setting will drive the staffing model. A full interdisciplinary team is usually appropriate for a large, tertiary care teaching hospital, while a part-time advance practice nurse with backup from colleagues may suffice for a small rural hospital or a long-term care setting. Programs are housed in a range of clinical subspecialties, including oncology, geriatrics, nursing, case management, and hospitalist programs, depending on the locus of leadership and administrative support.

Most programs are supported through diverse funding sources, including physician and nurse practitioner billing through insurers such as Medicare Part B, as well as hospital support (typically predicated on cost-avoidance analyses), foundation funding and other grants, and philanthropy from grateful families and citizens. The palliative care program will not generate a great deal of direct revenue for the hospital. However, it can sometimes cover its costs. More often, the program reduces costs for the hospital through cost avoidance.

How Are Programs Financed?

To help the team choose a realistic program size and structure, take into account:

- how much revenue the program can generate, given estimated patient volume;
- revenue from increased hospital capacity; and
- the cost savings from shorter length of stay and lower ancillary charges.

Detailed guidance on appropriate documentation and billing for palliative care physician services may be found at the Center to Advance Palliative Care website (www.capc.org). There, you will find information on how to complete financial analyses for the program, including how to estimate the following:

- program volume, both current and future;
- cost savings;
- hospital revenue enhancement;
- hospital billing revenues;
- revenues from physician billing;
- philanthropic donations; and
- costs.

What Is the Relationship between Hospice and Palliative Care Services?

Hospice and palliative care programs share similar goals; patients in either setting benefit from collaboration between the two. Palliative care programs based in hospital and community settings have led to increases in hospice referral rates and hospice length of stay, promoting continuity of palliative care and the intensive palliation and family support needed as death approaches. By coordinating with hospice services, palliative care services promote continuity of care, both through the course of an illness and across care settings.

What Are Common Barriers to Starting a Palliative Care Program?

By its very nature, institutional change often encounters barriers. Some commonly associated with developing a palliative care program are:

- educating clinicians and managers about the role of palliative care in severe chronic illness, not only for patients who are imminently dying, but also for those with illnesses that eventually lead to death;
- identifying patients who are appropriate for the program;
- overcoming physician fears about "losing" patients and patient fears of "giving up."

Physician concerns seem to be almost universal and revolve around the fear that they will be seen as "letting go" of patients or "giving up" on them. Although they have no reservations about referring patients to other specialists or units, they are often concerned that the palliative care group will be the "death squad" (as one hospitalist described it). Palliative care teams respond to these concerns in different ways, depending on existing personnel and staff organization. One group decided to keep its program as a consulting service rather than to set it up as a separate unit. On a consult basis, the team could come in, assess patients, and recommend treatments, all leaving the attending physician free to take their advice or not. Another group, which went ahead with a separate unit, found that the key to overcoming physician fears was to educate them about what was being offered. The palliative care physician had to reassure her colleagues that she was not trying to take over their patients or undermine their roles but to strengthen their ability to provide symptom management. A third group knew from the start that it did not want to add direct services but only to provide a vehicle to coordinate existing services, including pain management, critical care, and bioethics. This team wanted to be sure that the right clinicians were called in at appropriate times for consults.

Ways to overcome physician concerns include:

- recruiting clinicians with an interest and training in palliative care who have stature and respect in the community;
- relying on the hospital's existing relationship with hospice;
- turning to other programs, including your case management and discharge planning programs, chaplaincy, pain management, and geriatrics, for support as you build your case;
- using existing data about intensive care unit (ICU) or hospital lengths of stay, ventilator days, and pharmacy or ancillary costs per day to show the potential and actual financial benefits of your program;
- gathering support from trustees who are interested in palliative care.

Measures of Success

Once the program is up and running, you will need to track clinical and operational outcomes not only to conduct research and to justify your work but also to apply for grants and other funding. Programs usually collect data in several categories, primarily about patient outcomes, operational matters, patient satisfaction, and costs and utilization.

Patient data should include each patient's demographics, diagnosis, functional status, and the presence of advance care plans or do not resuscitate (DNR) orders. You will want outcome measures, such as pain and symptom control, advance care planning, referrals to hospice, number of hospitalizations and ICU admissions, transfers out of the ICU, palliative care interventions, referrals to spiritual support or bereavement services, and the place of death. Patient, family, and healthcare provider reports on their overall experience can also help measure the program's effect.

In terms of the program's operational measures, collect data about the volume and type of referrals, team workload, and the time between consult and improved symptoms. Finally, you will want to track financial data, especially the length of stay, ICU length of stay, the length of stay following the palliative care consult, and costs (in total, as well as direct and pharmacy costs), as listed below.

Clinical Outcomes

Clinical outcomes can include the following:

- decrease in severity of pain and other symptoms;
- number and type of palliative care interventionists and their effect;
- patient and family satisfaction;
- advance care planning discussion documentation in chart;
- number of DNR orders;
- transfers out of the ICU/hospital charges;
- hospice referrals.

Financial Effects

The financial effects of creating a palliative care program may be influenced by the following:

- length of stay (hospital and ICU);
- length of stay after palliative care consultation;

- total cost per day before and after consultation;
- pharmacy costs per day, before and after consultation.

PLAN FOR GROWTH

If you build it, usually, they will come. As other organizations have learned, palliative care programs tend to grow quickly and care for ever-increasing numbers of patients. The demand for these services will only continue to grow as the population ages. Teams must plan for success and prepare for increases in referrals and workloads to keep resources in line with demand. For example:

- plan prospectively for growth, and hire more staff as demand increases;
- avoid turning away referring physicians, if at all possible;
- consider enhancing skills for primary-care physicians so that only patients with advanced chronic conditions come for consultation;
- project and monitor program growth;
- revise the business plan to reflect the growth and other changes that can have significant implications for your program;
- maintain support to the leadership by tracking and reporting outcomes;
- remain highly responsive to the needs and circumstances of your organization;
- detect and address any quality problems that affect your program.

Once the program is working, do not forget to try QI tests that keep you focused on enhancing patient care.

TOOLS AND RESOURCES

- The Center to Advance Palliative Care
  1255 Fifth Avenue, Suite C-2
  New York, NY 10029
  212.201.2670
  http://www.capc.org
- Joint Commission on Accreditation of Healthcare
  Organizations (JCAHO), and the National Pharmaceutical
  Council. (2003, March). *Improving the Quality of Pain
  Management through Measurement and Action.* Retrieved
  January 20, 2006, from the JCAHO Web site
  http://www.jcaho.org/news+room/health+care+issues/
     pain_mono_jc.pdf
- National Consensus Project for Quality Palliative Care
  One Penn Center West, Suite 229
  Pittsburgh, PA 15276–0100
  http://www.nationalconsensusproject.org

REFERENCES

National Consensus Project for Quality Palliative Care. (2004). *The
   Development of Practice Guidelines 2004.* Retrieved January 20,
   2006, from the National Consensus Project Web site: http://www
   .nationalconsensusproject.org, accessed 08/10/05

World Health Organization (WHO). (1990). Cancer Pain Relief and Palliative Care. Report of WHO Expert Committee, Technical Series No. 804.
   Geneva: WHO.

Hospice Program Quality

In This Chapter

- Identifying opportunities
- Making improvements—not just changes and more paperwork
- Practical guidelines for quality improvement in hospice settings

Hospices, like other healthcare organizations, may soon be required by federal regulations to focus on quality improvement (QI) efforts and demonstrate whether they are effective in improving patient care. This chapter describes QI strategies particular to hospice settings, which may also be useful in meeting the proposed Medicare "conditions of participation" (42 CFR Part 418, 2005).

Team Hospice

A community hospice in an urban area undertook a project to improve the care of people recently admitted to hospice. Complaints from patients and interdisciplinary team (IDT) members pointed to problems with gaps in timeliness and in completeness of information exchanged between admissions staff and the other members of the IDT. Patients were not being seen promptly for follow-up of identified problems and were left with physical and/or emotional discomfort for too long. The admissions nurse phoned reports to the rest of the IDT. Reports had no consistent format and were time consuming to record and listen to; this resulted in IDT members sometimes missing problems that needed prompt or immediate attention. After listening to the admission reports, staff decided that scripting reports would not only help IDT members track information, but would also help the nurse write admission notes more efficiently.

Identifying the Problem and Setting an Aim Statement

By the end of the project, your QI activity will have an important outcome for patients and their loved ones. The National Hospice and Palliative Care Organization (NHPCO) groups major outcomes as follows:

- self-determined life closure for all patients;
- safe and comfortable dying for all patients;
- effective grieving for the patient and the family.

The National Institutes of Health (NIH) State of the Science Conference Statement on Improving End-of-Life Care (December 2004, http://consensus.nih.gov/2004/2004EndOfLifeCareSOS024html.htm) lists examples of broad outcome domains that are important indicators of quality end-of-life experience for the dying person: "physical or psychological symptoms, social relationships, spiritual or philosophical beliefs, hopes, expectations and meaning, satisfaction, economic considerations, and caregiver and family experience."

These domains may give you an idea of where to start in QI. What problems occur in your hospice program that result in patient or family complaints, regulatory deficiencies, or care outcomes that you wish were better? Monitoring program measures on a continuous basis helps you know which problems are growing and which areas need attention. This data is often available to you from reports you complete for audits, regulatory agencies, NHPCO, or others. Pick an area where you see room for improvement and discuss how the improvement will benefit patients, families, and staff.

Here are some questions to get you started.

- Does the admissions process occur in a timely manner, do you receive an adequate diagnosis from the referral source, and do you quickly have an adequate initial care plan?
- Are patients referred to hospice "too late?"
- Is pain resolved within 24 hours of admission?
- Are depression, constipation, and other symptoms recognized and treated appropriately?
- Are patients' and their families' spiritual and psychological needs considered and respected?
- Is the do not resuscitate (DNR) order and healthcare proxy available and complete?
- Are patients' wishes regarding end-of-life treatment documented? Has the patient said where he or she would prefer to die?
- Do patients' families have sufficient help with direct services and support?
- Are patients spared unnecessary transfers to the hospital?
- Is there confusion about the roles and responsibilities with staff in nursing homes?
- Is palliative sedation done in a timely manner, and is it done with adequate diagnosis?
- Does staff have a specific timeframe for responding to family calls?
- Do all patients reach their acceptable pain level within a specific time period?

- Are there medication errors?
- Are preventable falls occurring?
- Are patients' wishes being followed?
- Is there adequate backup for hospice staff in the home?

Your answers to these questions will point you to areas for QI. Figure 13.1 offers a way to envision how to move from identifying a problem to making changes that will improve patient care.

Looking at the domains and the list of common problems may calm some of the "data blues" that people sometimes experience with QI activities since many items in the lists have built-in outcome measures. For example, the National Data Set Survey or the Family Evaluation of Hospice Care Survey (available only to NHPCO members) match up well. Recognizing the priority areas for improvement depends on an ongoing assessment of performance and on staying abreast of benchmarks and best practices as they develop.

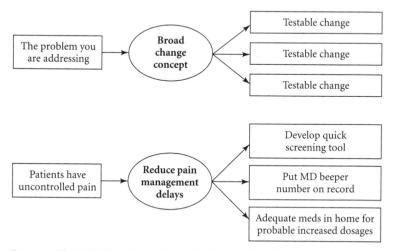

FIGURE 13.1 Thinking about change, both generally and for pain management

Setting an Aim Statement

Your aim statement will tell people how your work will benefit the patient: what outcome do you hope to achieve by making changes? Once you have an aim, you will want to focus on measuring, analyzing, and tracking one or more related quality indicators. For instance, if you decide to work on ensuring that all newly admitted patients have acceptable pain relief, you may use an aim such as "All newly admitted patients will have acceptable pain relief by the end of the second day" as your quality indicator (see Chapter 2 to help you construct your aim statement so that it contains all four elements: what will improve, for whom, by how much, and when).

Do not settle for a small change; after learning the model for improvement, you can expect to have big results. Put that expectation in your aim statement. Perhaps you have chosen an aim to have pain relieved in each person in hospice at home by the end of the second day; stretch that aim to have pain and all other physical symptoms relieved or addressed within 24 hours of admission. Or, if you are sure you can make an improvement for 14% of a certain population, aim to spread the improvement to 94% of that population. Once you have figured out how to make a difference for a small number of people, spreading it to a larger population is much easier—indeed, you already know what works. The QI model is a powerful way to make powerful improvements; don't sell yourself short by aiming too low.

Team Hospice

After reviewing their current practices, Team Hospice decided to focus their QI based on Medicare's proposed regulations.

Aim: By July of next year, 100% of patients in Urban Hospice will have problems, issues, and opportunities (PIOs) identified on admission, and acute PIOs will be assessed and addressed on admission with follow-up by the close of business of the second hospice day.

What will improve: *Acute PIOs will be addressed on admission and followed up by the close of the second hospice day.*
By when: *By July of next year.*
By how much: *One hundred percent.*
For whom: *Patients in Urban Hospice.*

Target Populations

You probably want all of the patients you serve to benefit from your QI projects, and eventually they will, if it is appropriate for them. Pick a particular small number of patients to begin your project. Some projects focus on newly admitted patients to the home-care services, others focus on people with certain diagnoses. Once your target population has benefited from your change, then you can move to include more patients in your change process. You will also want to make sure that there are enough people in your target population so that you can easily measure the success of your changes. If your hospice only has two patients with amyotrophic lateral sclerosis (ALS) each year, for instance, you might want to include a larger category of patients, including those with ALS. Looking at only two cases per year will never be enough to show you whether a change is really an improvement.

Choosing a Team

The key in choosing a team is to consider all of the staff whose work affects the targeted patient or issue. A pain relief project will require medical and nursing staff, as well as a pharmacist who may act as a consultant to the team. A team looking at overall patient comfort may include home-care aides and a social worker or chaplain so that no area is overlooked. Three to five members are enough for the core team, and others can be invited when their input, support, or good ideas are needed. Be sure to include senior leadership on the team, if possible. Otherwise, keep them informed and up to date. There may be occasions when you will need their assistance, and that is *not* the ideal time to start telling them about your project.

MEASURING YOUR SUCCESS

Look at what you already have for quality indicators before adding more paperwork to your existence. Arguably, your intended improvement will affect a patient or family outcome that is already tracked in your charting. If so, use that data before inventing another way to monitor. Pain scores, for example, are already part of the patient's record. Times and amounts of medication, number of visits, and number of phone calls are all there, waiting to become data for your QI project. Another potential source of data for tracking can be found in your family/patient satisfaction/outcome survey. General satisfaction is not often a good outcome measure because it is insensitive to the quality of care. The NHPCO After-Death Family Survey asks families to report specific events and perceptions and is more useful in guiding improvements than merely tallying satisfaction.

TEAM HOSPICE

Using the aim statement of Team Hospice, the measures will be as follows.

Aim: By July of next year, 100% of patients in Urban Hospice will have PIOs identified on admission, and acute PIOs will be assessed and addressed on admission, with follow-up by the close of business of the second hospice day.

> **Outcome Measure:** *The percentage of patients for whom the electronic hospice record reflects that all acute PIOs are recorded and addressed by the end of the second hospice day, divided by the number of patients admitted each month.*
>
> **Process Measure 1:** *The percentage of admitted patients who have their identified PIOs communicated to the IDT within 24 hours of admission via report form that is documented in the record.*
>
> **Process Measure 2:** *The percentage of staff using admission forms to give an oral report on the day of admission.*
>
> **Adverse-Effect Measure:** *The percentage of admission report users who tell the team leader that the oral report wastes time.*

TIME SERIES GRAPHS

A visual display of your outcomes and the progress you are making toward the goal is a powerful QI tool. You can use time series graphs to plot the success of your outcome goals over time. Time series charts are a very concise and clear way of showing your process and your results. Team Hospice used the following time series graph (see Figure 13.2) to track their results.

IDENTIFYING AND TESTING CHANGES

TEAM HOSPICE

After much brainstorming, team members at Urban Hospice identified the following changes to try out to improve patient care in their organization.

- *They developed a new admissions report form to exchange information. Team members initially developed this form and*

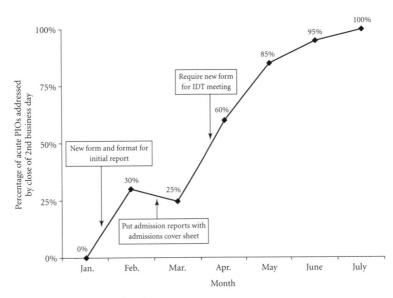

FIGURE 13.2 Team Hospice

later fine tuned it with the help of key staff, including a medical director, a nurse manager, a chaplain, and a social worker.

- *They summarized admissions reports with one-page cover sheets. The administrative assistant was responsible for accomplishing this.*

- *The team also began using the admissions reports for the IDT meeting, which helped the meeting run more smoothly and efficiently.*

Reviewing where the gaps are in your hospice service and learning from others will help you decide which change or changes you need to make to improve care. If a tool exists that you think will help, use it;

do not waste time inventing a new one. For ideas for change, consult the chapters in this book for topic areas that interest you, keep reading professional journals, and attend professional meetings. The NHPCO standards can provide further assistance.

Introduce a new tool or procedure on a small number of patients, and then see if you are getting the desired effects. If not, you can adapt the tool or the procedure until it is most useful to you, and then you can begin to use it in other areas.

Start the changes with people who are supportive of your idea. For example, it may be that one nurse uses the Edmonton Symptom Assessment Scale with the patients assigned to her care, and once she sees the scale's benefit for her patients, she will encourage other nurses to use it, too, and thus can help spread the change to all nurses.

TEAM HOSPICE

Admissions nurses at Urban Hospice were asked to use the new admissions report. Initially, use of the report hovered around 30%, with a spike of 70% after a training session. Using the form seemed to depend on the team leader encouraging admissions staff to use it. To test that observation, a 10-question survey of all team members asked for their feedback about using the form and suggestions for improving it.

Three issues arose from that survey:

1. *Forms were not readily available to use and not part of the admissions packet;*

2. *Admissions nurses did not believe that using the form made a difference to patient care;*

3. *The nurses' stories about the people they met during the admissions were left untold. The rich descriptions of patients' families, which have been prominent in the history of hospice nursing, were put on the back burner by the admissions report. Admissions nurses and hospice-service nurses felt that they had lost*

something important in the process. They found it important to be able to tell patients' stories, even though they saw the value of the streamlined report.

To address the needs of the team to record patient stories and get support for their difficult work, the team decided to have quarterly meetings and more frequent educational/support group meetings. More and more people began using the report form with less and less effort. The admissions report form has now been in use for two years; it is used 100% of the time for admissions reports and to introduce patients in IDT team meetings. Completing the form is now in the admissions nurse job description and is addressed in staff orientation as a standard hospice policy.

Hospice programs promise patients and their families unusually comprehensive, high-quality, reliable services. It is especially important to ensure expert skills and assiduous attention since the patient will probably not live long enough for you to correct any shortcomings. Quality improvement processes can be a strong method to ensure high performance.

Tools and Resources

- 42 CFR Part 418. (2005). Medicare and Medicaid Programs: Proposed Conditions of Participation; Proposed Rule. Retrieved August 9, 2006, from the Center for Medicare and Medicaid Web site,
http://www.cms.hhs.gov/quarterlyproviderupdates/Downloads/CMS3844P.pdf
- Hallenbeck, J. (2005). *Ten Simple Things You Can Do to Access Hospice and Palliative Care Resources.* Retrieved August 9, 2006, from Hallenbeck's blog on Growth House, Inc.

http://growthhouse.typepad.com/james_hallenbeck/2005/08/
  ten_simple_thin.html

- Henderson, M., Hanson, L., & Reynolds, K. (Eds.). (2003).
  Flacker mortality scale. In *Improving Nursing Home Care of the
  Dying*. New York: Springer.
- Edmonton Symptom Assessment Scale
  http://www.promotingexcellence.org/chicago/downloads/
  ucp13.pdf
- National Hospice and Palliative Care Organization
  http://www.nhpco.org
- National Institutes of Health (NIH). (2004, December). State
  of the Science Conference Statement on Improving End-of-
  Life Care. Retrieved January 20, 2006, from the NIH Web site:
  http:// consensus.nih.gov/2004/2004EndOfLifeCareSOS024
  html.htm

14

End-of-Life Care, Spiritual Support, and Bereavement

In This Chapter

- Understanding the importance of the last few days and hours of life
- Improving psychosocial, spiritual, and bereavement support to patients and loved ones
- Improving support and bereavement services for healthcare providers and staff

One of the many ways in which healthcare providers can assist patients, their families, and their providers in experiencing a "good death" is to help them prepare for the event and to provide facts, advice, and support to the family and friends of those who are near death. The time spent living with fatal illness is important to patients and their loved ones because it offers a time to strengthen connections, build memories, and shape the final days.

In the end, when families tell others about a loved one's death, they will be grateful if the patient was not in pain—and they will certainly remember the kind nurse from the night shift, the transfer orderly who made sure the patient was comfortable, or the nursing aide who treated the patient with such respect and concern. So, this is the story that you want your patients' survivors to tell: that the dying was comfortable, that the staff was kind and thoughtful, and that the end was as good as it could have been and respectful of the patient's values and preferences.

Too often there are other stories to tell: the loneliness of a death-bed vigil; the isolation of living with a life-limiting disease; the medical "system" that was impossible to navigate; and the staff who did not seem to care. Remember, too, that your staff members have emotional, psychosocial, and spiritual needs as they care for patients. Staff in all healthcare settings, perhaps especially CNAs, can become attached to the patient and the patient's family. For some residents with no one, the staff can become like family. Quality improvement (QI) teams often find that staff members need time to acknowledge a death and honor the patient's life.

Quality improvement teams find that even small changes in end-of-life care, bereavement, and spiritual support usually lead to an improvement. Providing a place for families to freshen up or spend time alone while keeping vigil with a loved one is quite effective in showing that the organization truly cares. Offering to bring in a member of the clergy who can speak to a patient or family member's particular beliefs and needs is a way to promote spiritual care. Making sure that families have easy access to one clinical team member for questions or concerns means the organization cares about keeping the family fully informed. Providing volunteers to help families through the dying process can be a meaningful contribution (see Chapter 10 on dementia care, Chapter 6 on caregiving, and Chapter 7 on continuity and transfers for more details). And, following up with family after the death of the patient to see how they are doing is an important basic improvement.

Research indicates that end-of-life patients and families fear pain, dependency, and loneliness and that they desire personal control over the circumstances and time of death. In our work, we have learned that patients and families often seek similar things in the final phase of life.

End-of-Life Issues Often Important to Patients and Caregivers

- Accurate and timely information about the patient's illness and what to expect during this last phase of life.
- Good medical care for and the maintenance of the dignity of the patient, including pain and other symptom management and good personal care of the patient.
- Respectful communication from healthcare providers and the involvement of patients and caregivers in clinical decision-making.
- Time for spiritual and emotional preparation for the end of life, including participation in decision-making, the opportunity to discuss personal fears and concerns with a trusted person, making peace with themselves and others, and saying good-bye.
- Having the dying person's financial affairs in order, and making plans for any dependents, including disabled family members and pets.
- Referral to facility and community resources to address needs and concerns.
- Attention to patients' and caregivers' psychosocial, spiritual, and bereavement needs before and after death.

Teams often need to customize generic bereavement materials to specific end-of-life populations (e.g., dementia patients rather than cancer patients, children rather than adults, or atheists rather than religious believers) and offer the right information to the right caregivers. Teams have also found that clergy, social workers, and volunteers are very good bereavement staff and that trained volunteers can conduct the initial bereavement follow-up calls effectively and compassionately. The guiding rule for materials used in these QI projects is "the simpler the better." That is, simple, straightforward materials and assessment tools proved to be the most useful. For example, even sending a listing of available grief-support resources in the community immediately following the death had a positive effect on caregivers. More information can be sent a few weeks or months later, including a follow-up call to ensure caregiver or staff adjustment. We have found that telephone follow-ups add a personal touch that families appreciate.

IDENTIFYING THE PROBLEM AND SETTING AN AIM

TEAM SCHMIDT

Schmidt Nursing Home wanted to improve the quality of life and death for residents in the advanced stages of life-limiting illnesses. A core QI team decided to conduct after-death interviews with families of residents who had died in the last six months, as well as with other residents with whom the resident had been friends. The team turned to dining room companions, and also talked to CNAs and other staff who had had direct, daily contact with recently deceased residents, to learn more about what had happened and what the residents and staff wanted to do in the future. In the course of this process, the team identified many problems, including the following.

- *Residents talked about their fear of dying alone—either because family could not make it to the home in time or because they had "no one" left who would keep vigil for them.*
- *Residents wanted to be notified when someone died; instead, though staff never openly talked about it, they usually heard through the grapevine or pieced it together by themselves because all the doors on a hall were closed as a body was removed.*
- *Staff members were upset when residents died and wished that they had a way to honor the dead.*
- *Staff who had been reassigned to another floor still wanted a*

chance to say good-bye to a dying resident and the resident's family.

- *Staff did not know what to do when they came across a deceased resident's personal belongings or arts-and-crafts projects: they could not just throw things away; but at the same time, they could not hold on to everything.*
- *Bereaved families were upset when a final bill came addressed to the deceased person.*
- *Families were surprised, and even hurt, when they didn't hear from floor nurses or Schmidt's medical director when their loved one died.*

Team Schmidt met to discuss the findings. Everyone seemed to have an idea that could create a change for the better. However, they were not sure if they understood the family members' priorities. They decided to conduct small focus-group discussions with some family caregivers whose loved ones had died within the last six months. They also sought feedback on the Continuing Care Program (home health, hospice, and long-term palliative care services). From these activities, the team looked for gaps in care, especially the ways in which the patient or caregiver was left dangling for something more—more care and more options.

Like Team Schmidt, once you start looking for trouble, you are likely to find it everywhere. Do not feel overwhelmed. Other groups have run into similar situations and have found that as they improve on one particular element of care, other elements seem to come along for the ride. You need to think through the problems you identify, rank them, and create a coherent set of activities with which to address them. For example, is your team doing well in other aspects of advanced illness and end-of-life care, such as having current advance care plans (ACPs) in the patients' records and accessible to all members of the care team?

(See Chapter 3 on ACP for more details.) Are you providing institutional support for families and clinical staff? (See Chapter 6 on caring for caregivers.) Are you doing a good job in caring for the dying patient? Are families and staff left to drift after the death of a patient or resident? If so, you may need to focus on bereavement support.

Before you can improve care, you need to learn more about the issues that patients, families, and staff are facing. Each group of patients and caregivers may have different issues that need attention (for more details, see Chapter 1, Figure 1.1, on trajectories). Obtaining baseline data from the caregivers of current and former patients of your program may help your team brainstorm what is needed. For example, follow-up phone calls to even a few (10–20) caregivers of recently deceased patients to determine how the caregiver is managing, what problems they are facing, and how they viewed the patient's end-of-life experience may point out problems. Surveys of staff regarding issues they see in the care of patients at the end of life can illuminate areas for improvement for staff, as well as patients and families. Once you have identified the key issues that need attention, settle on at least one aim, and figure out how you will measure your improvement efforts.

TEAM SCHMIDT

After a month of brainstorming, survey/focus-group data analysis, and a few meetings, Team Schmidt developed four aim statements.

Aim 1: *Within three months, 80% of family members whose relative died in Schmidt Nursing Home will have received a condolence card and a bereavement packet of educational materials on grief and loss, and they will be made aware of bereavement resources and grief support groups in the community.*

Aim 2: *Within six months, 100% of "at risk of death" residents with no family members available, who state that they do not want to die alone, will have an "Angel at the Bedside" (a volunteer* *trained to sit with a dying person) assigned and working with the resident within 48 hours of identification.*

Aim 3: *Within eight months, 80% of surviving family members will say they received bereavement services and that they were either helpful or very helpful.*

Aim 4: *Within eight months, 80% of "at risk of dying" residents will be provided with enhanced palliative care services through the end of life.*

These aim statements were grounded by the following criteria.

What will improve: *Access to bereavement services for families of patients who die.*

By how much: *80% (rather than current happenstance referrals).*

By when: *Within eight months.*

For whom: *Families of Schmidt Nursing Home whose relative died in the facility.*

Choosing a Team

Shared leadership frames the work of rapid-cycle QI. Your team should include people who will affect or be affected by the interventions. Most teams include a champion (usually a physician or nurse practitioner) with clinical expertise, a person who will shoulder the day-to-day tasks, someone who understands QI, and a leader with the administrative clout to push for the resources to make it happen. Be sure that you choose teammates who are open to new ideas, committed to change, and supportive of your goal to improve care.

Team Schmidt

Team Schmidt knew that they needed help and wanted to include people with specific expertise. Their team already consisted of the be-

reavement coordinator, a music therapist, a chaplain, the nurse manager for the long-term care unit, and a social worker. The team decided to ask the volunteer coordinator from an affiliated senior living facility and a volunteer coordinator from a local hospice organization to join the project. They knew that their planned intervention would require volunteers to make it work, and the affiliated senior living facility and service organization seemed like good sources for compassionate volunteers. In addition, they began to work with the social worker to develop a training program for volunteers. They added a nurse from the local hospice, a family member whose relative had died six months prior, and the nurse practitioner. They also made plans to invite the chief executive officer to their next meeting so that one of their senior leaders would be sympathetic and supportive of the changes that they knew they had to make. Eventually, they called on the local hospice for its expertise in care for imminently dying people, and they asked the hospice's chaplain to help them develop resources for keeping vigil.

MEASURING SUCCESS

Your team needs to decide what data to collect, the person who will be responsible for it, and how often you will collect it (see Chapter 2 on QI basics). Depending on how big your patient population is, you might want to sample patients to get an unbiased yet manageable data size. You also need to figure out how you will display your data: daily, weekly, every other week, monthly, or quarterly. Be sure to collect enough data to build a case (or to see where an improvement is not working).

Although it is hard to measure directly a patient's or caregiver's sense of anxiety, fear, or isolation, you can make proxy measures that give you a feel for whether the change that you are trying is an improvement. In the case of Schmidt's third aim statement, the measure can be quantified by the following.

> *Process Measure: The percentage of families who received information about bereavement services after a resident's death.*
>
> *Outcome Measure: Of families who received bereavement services, the percentage who found these services helpful or very helpful.*
>
> *Adverse-Effect Measure: The families who report that follow-up calls were distressing or unwanted.*

You may need to revise your aim so that it focuses on something you can quantify and track. In any case, not all changes are an improvement and the only way to know for sure is to measure your progress. Following are some end-of-life spiritual and bereavement measures.

Process Measures

- Dying patients/residents whose treatment preferences are incorporated into an ACP and reviewed quarterly.
- Targeting of patients with end-of-life symptoms and signs that are routinely assessed and documented in the medical record.
- Volunteers are trained and available to sit with dying patients.
- Bereaved family members are referred to appropriate grief counseling.
- Bereaved family caregivers who attend bereavement services.
- Bereaved caregivers who receive a follow-up telephone call within three months of a patient's death.
- Bereaved caregivers who receive a follow-up bereavement assessment based on the three-month follow-up call.
- Bereaved caregivers with significant psychosocial problems who receive a home counseling visit and referral to community resources.

- Staff who participate in facility-sponsored bereavement support services, such as monthly remembrance groups, patient funerals, or quarterly nursing home services.

TELLING YOUR STORY: TIME SERIES GRAPH

TEAM SCHMIDT

To measure progress, Team Schmidt decided to chart how many of its target patients died alone (without a family or staff member) in their nursing home. To make sure that their results were not biased, they tallied only those patients whose deaths were expected within at least eight hours. Data were charted monthly (see Figures 14.1 and 14.2).

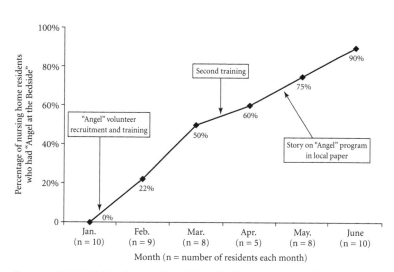

FIGURE 14.1 Within six months, 100% of residents at risk of dying who state that they do not want to die alone will have an "Angel at the Bedside" (a volunteer trained to sit with a dying person).

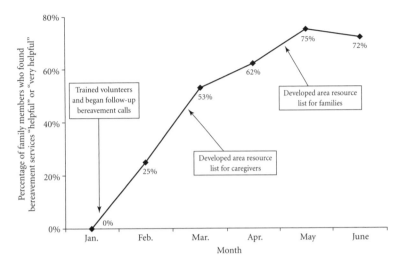

FIGURE 14.2   Within eight months, 80% of surviving family members where death occurred in the Schmidt Nursing Home will say they received bereavement services that were "helpful" or "very helpful."

IDENTIFYING AND TESTING CHANGES

TEAM SCHMIDT

The team tested its project with imminently dying patients on one floor, relying on volunteers from the hospice's grief-support program to keep vigil. Because so many people had stated their fears of dying alone, the team assumed that the presence of another human being would make a difference. To find the real effects of their work, the team began to survey the bereaved family members and staff. These results showed that families felt comforted by the promise that their loved ones would not die alone. Over the course of six months, the team had received a half-dozen letters from grateful family members. Staff also reported on how important it was to them to maintain a human presence for these patients.

In the first few weeks of implementing the changes, the team felt disappointed because some families felt overwhelmed by both the deaths of their loved ones and the bereavement activities of the bereavement QI team. Was the team helping? The team reviewed the first few months of data, including informal discussions with "overwhelmed" caregivers, and decided that they would simplify their mailed materials and expand their telephone follow-up tools to maintain accurate identification of problems with grief and ensure consistent follow-up to services for the families. In addition, they decided to focus on how well the facility addressed dying patients' needs, such as pain and symptom management, care consistent with the patients' stated wishes, and reduced or eliminated transfers of dying residents to the hospital when appropriate. Next, they decided to tackle the issues of patient comfort and unnecessary transfers.

Individual counseling services are helpful when an individual caregiver faces a particularly challenging event or period of time in the disease or after the death of a patient. Support group interventions provide caregivers and staff with an opportunity to realize that they are not alone and to discuss common problems and fears with other caregivers. Research suggests that support group interventions provide needed information about diseases and practical and psychological issues, as well as informal support networking for caregivers who are receptive to this kind of assistance. Monthly or quarterly memorial services for all families of patients who died in a particular program facility and for staff who worked with the patients are often highly valued in the bereavement process.

Following are some examples of five general areas of support that teams can use to develop excellent care for the time near death and for spiritual and bereavement support for their patients, families, and staff.

Communication with Families

- Listen to patients and their families, provide time for discussion of concerns and fears, and invite questions.
- Do not allow interruptions when meeting with families concerning care plan development or updates.
- Provide accurate, timely, and complete information to patients, families, and staff.
- Speak honestly and sensitively with patients, families, and staff about each patient's situation.
- Learn to talk comfortably with families, staff, and residents about death and dying.
- Ensure periodic review of patient and family preferences for end-of-life care.

Communication with Healthcare Clinicians and Staff in Other Settings

- Provide complete patient information on "hand off" or transfer to new settings, including patient status, care wishes, and treatment plan.
- Reduce unnecessary transfers of patients who want to "stay home" in the facility until death.
- Provide timely transfer of information across providers when transfer is appropriate.
- Standardize forms for transfer of uniform information among partner facilities in region.
- Use interdisciplinary team (IDT) management as a standard of care.
- Create uniform forms and protocols for transfer among local providers.

Emotional, Psychosocial, and Spiritual Support
of Patients and Families

- Show evidence of the provision of compassionate, hopeful, respectful, and comfortable care to patients and family members.
- Establish evidence-based, systematic programs, services, and care protocols for end-of-life care.
- Adopt culturally and individually appropriate language, materials, and services.
- Provide trained "Angels at the Bedside" for vigils for residents without family or to supplement family visits.
- Provide an end-of-life care volunteer to help families through the dying process.
- Assess and respond to the emotional and/or spiritual needs of patients, caregivers, or staff.

Provider Access and Fear of Abandonment

- Be available when patients or families have questions or want to talk, and allow patients and caregivers the opportunity to express concerns.
- Ensure that patients and their families will receive the kind of care desired by helping to find what they need.
- Provide excellent, evidence-based, interdisciplinary deathbed palliative care.
- Reassure patients and families that the patient will not be abandoned at the end of life, mostly by ensuring continuity of clinicians.
- Address ethical issues in end-of-life care, such as ventilator withdrawal, tube feeding, and transfers.
- Provide hospitality carts and private spaces for families keeping vigils.

TEAM SCHMIDT

After seeing that the initial changes led to improvements for residents, Team Schmidt looked for ways to make the changes part of their institutional culture. Because Schmidt was part of a statewide long-term care corporation, its work began to spread to other nursing homes in their system, first by word-of-mouth, then through the corporate newsletter. The director of nursing visited six allied facilities to give presentations on spirituality and end-of-life programs. The team also began to involve the chaplain routinely in working with end-of-life patients and families as a way to give health-related information to families. The chaplain had contact numbers for nursing units and administrators printed on the back of his business card which he could give to each patient and family with whom he visited. Team Schmidt amended the nursing home's family survey to include questions asking surviving family members about their perceptions of their relatives during their final days in the facility.

TOOLS AND RESOURCES

- Grief Steps: Bereavement Support Services for Families in Transition
  http://www.griefsteps.com
- Open Directory: Health, Mental Health, Grief, Loss, and Bereavement Support Resources
  http://dmoz.org
- Bereavement Services: Training and Support Services for Professionals Who Care for Bereaved Families
  http://www.bereavementprograms.com
- Your local hospice(s), churches, and social work agencies

15

Beyond Quality Improvement
Policy Improvement

You have done everything you can to improve the care of seriously ill and dying patients in your care setting—but you can see that so much more remains to be done. You have transformed the lives and deaths of 30–40 patients, but you want to do the same for thousands of patients. But how? What an overwhelming challenge!

Or is it? In fact, you can do a great deal to improve care of the dying, not only in your facility but in facilities around the country. Sound daunting? Sure, if you wanted to intervene personally in each case. But how about intervening through public policy—through the laws, regulations, and traditions that keep us locked into our usual routine? Perhaps you could work at a broader level to change public policies that influence how the healthcare and social services systems manage care for people with advanced chronic illnesses and those facing life-limiting illnesses. Healthcare policy influences so much of how we die, from where we die to what we pay for services. By changing public policies, we can change how things happen; we can push for coordinated care across multiple settings and providers, for swift and appropriate management of symptoms, or for the much-needed, home-based support for patients and their families. And you—ordinary citizen, healthcare professional or paraprofessional—have the power to influence all these policies. Use your voice, your intellect, your vote, and your profession. In short, advocate to change behavior and change attitudes!

This chapter touches on policies that affect those with a life-limiting chronic illness, those at the final phase of life, and what you can do to change them. To learn more, we recommend that you read Joanne Lynn's book *Sick to Death and Not Going to Take It Anymore!* You can also take special note of issues being pursued by professional and consumer interest groups, such as the American Society of Clinical Oncologists, the American Geriatrics Society, or the local Alzheimer's Association. While groups are likely to follow pressing issues that may focus on their own specific interests, such as physician fee schedules or prescription drug coverage, they may need your encouragement to add end-of-life issues to their agenda. In some cases, you will find that the group is actually working at various levels of government in ways that will advance your own agenda about improving care at the final phase of life.

How We Die

When we talk about growing old, most Americans imagine that we will enjoy a secure retirement, good health, and a quick exit. We think we will somehow escape the problems that plagued our own parents or grandparents—and, in a way, we will. But instead of dying young, from an acute illness, most of us will grow old while accumulating one or more chronic diseases. Years ago, these diseases would have killed us in a few months or weeks. Now, however, we will live with these ailments for several years, growing progressively worse and increasingly disabled. While we enjoy an increased life expectancy (now averaging 77 years for women, 73 years for men), we will also live with increasing illnesses. Our final years may prove painful and difficult, especially if played out with the current healthcare system. The so-called golden years often prove to be the leaden years, with families overwhelmed by the emotional and financial burdens of care.

As currently designed, our healthcare and community social services systems are not organized to meet the needs of the large and growing number of people facing this long period of progressive illness and disability. In the current system, it is often easier to get open-heart surgery than it is to get a bedpan. For the very old and frail, the healthcare system does not spend much time or resources on cures; these are mostly quick and cheap, when they are available at all. Instead, for this part of our lives, healthcare is no longer about treatment and cure, but about helping people to live with implacable illnesses. A few of these conditions are stable, and many are progressive but not life-threatening. However, each of us will eventually live with a set of conditions that are, taken together, progressively worsening and eventually fatal.

And the news just does not get better. Over the next 30 years, the number of Americans living to 85 years or older will double, from 4.2 million in 2000 to almost 9 million by 2030. They will take their health problems with them: those who reach their eighth decade will likely live with several disabling chronic conditions and with increasing frailty. At the same time, care for this population is increasingly expensive, and the supply of professional and family caregivers is dwindling.

The only good news is that you—along with thousands of other healthcare professionals involved in quality improvement (QI) programs—want to change the situation for your patients and their families. And those changes can reverberate for other patients in other settings. With prodding, the healthcare system will change, too. It has adapted to demographic changes before, and it can do so again. But adapting requires learning to see advanced chronic illness and the end of life in new ways and revamping the healthcare system so as to deliver and finance the necessary services.

For now, hospice is our best model for what could be. Indeed, one half of Americans with cancer use hospice care for at least a short time before dying. However, for most of the time when people live with serious chronic illness that will end in death, hospice care is not an option. For much of this time, people live with chronic illness, that indistinct zone which has no specific care-delivery system and that leaves them to manage mostly on their own. Some changes, however, are underway. Despite our cultural, and perhaps our universally human, distaste for the facts of finitude and death, we are gradually coming to grips with the reality of disability in old age and the necessary truth of serious illness and death. Just 30 years ago, most hospital staff attempted resuscitation on every person whose heart stopped. Now, only a small minority, mostly patients who might actually benefit, have resuscitation attempted. In fact, the U.S. Preventive Services Task Force has started including some "upper limits" on the ages at which screening tests make sense (see http://www.ahrq.gov/clinic/uspstfab.htm).

But real improvement will require real change, not just a change in the words we use or the limits that we set. Instead, what is needed is a change of focus and direction in how we view the time near the final phase of life, both for dying people and for their loved ones.

THE WAY TO GO: TRAJECTORY-BASED SYSTEMS OF CARE FOR THE DYING

We cannot design a healthcare system to suit the needs of each dying person; instead, we need to find ways to tailor what we know about end-of-life care so that it works for most people, most of the time, in most situations. As it is, we rely on a rather ad hoc approach to care, piecing together what we know and using what we can. In the end, families often feel that they are lucky if they get good care—and not that they should have received good care or that they expect good care in the first place—only that, for one person, care came together in a way that made sense. The trouble with this is that for many people care does not come together, and their final days are spent in suffering and fear while anxious family members wait helplessly.

What might work better? We could build the care system around common trajectories of dying, matching care to the size and characteristics of a specific population and its predictable needs. In the introduction, we described three trajectories of dying that seem to cover the ways in which most adults eventually die. Right now, we care for people based on their particular diagnoses on a given day, with care shifting from one setting to another, often in response to an acute illness or exacerbation. We might do better to expect a particular course across time and to anticipate needs.

The three trajectories are roughly sequential in the ages afflicted, with fatal cancers peaking around age 65, fatal chronic organ system failures roughly a decade later, and frailty and dementia afflicting mostly those who live past their mid-80s. As science and public health more reliably prevent or delay the onset of cancer, emphysema, and heart disease, the proportion of the population facing the third course will increase.

This approach of conceiving of the challenge of care for the final phase of life as a problem of system design reflects a very different concept than just relying on patient autonomy. Important as advance directives (ADs) are, the core problem is not just patient and physician decision-making. In fact, we cannot assume or assure that good care arises from prudent choices by individual doctors and patients. Rather, such care will come only when the care system is designed to serve the vast majority of patients "on autopilot." That is, right things will happen for almost all patients because the right actions have been built into the system and have become a routine part of care.

PRIORITY CARE NEEDS FOR THE THREE ILLNESS TRAJECTORIES

For Short Period of Evident Decline (Mostly Cancer), Consider:

- adapting services to rapid changes in the patient;
- controlling symptoms;
- providing support for families, including training, respite, and counseling through bereavement;

- ensuring continuity of the clinical team;
- offering opportunities for life closure and completion.

*For Chronic Illnesses with Intermittent Exacerbations and
Sudden Dying (Mostly Organ System Failure), Consider:*

- preventing exacerbations and providing early treatment;
- planning for urgent situations;
- making decisions about the benefits of low-yield treatments;
- mobilizing services to the home;
- preparing families for sudden death;
- life closure and completion.

For Slow Dwindling (Mostly Frailty and Dementia), Consider:

- fostering caregiver endurance, loyalty, and reliability;
- providing long-term personal care services and supervision;
- helping family caregivers to find meaning and avoid severe
  emotional and financial burdens;
- avoiding undesired prolongation of life;
- keeping skin intact;
- finding pleasurable moments that patients enjoy;
- attending to the need for life closure and completion.

Hospice represents a system of care that reliably can serve patients
who will die quickly; that is, those who have a high likelihood of death
within six months. Even though the Medicare hospice benefit is now
unlimited, the patient must continue to have a short prognosis to
qualify; thus, it does not serve people who live beyond their prognosis after a persistently unpredictable course. No strategy is currently
available, for example, that would optimally serve most heart-failure
patients through the years when they can be treated successfully,
which is also the unpredictable period during which they are likely
to die. Most advanced chronic conditions, including heart failure,

have a course that is simply too unpredictable, and good services cannot be put in place on a case-by-case basis or only for those very likely to die soon.

There is so much yet to be learned about optimal care for people living with fatal disease. This must have been the state of science regarding heart disease 50 years ago, when most of the "science" was expert opinion and much of it was inadequate or even in error. Surely, as the huge population of Baby Boomers reaches old age and death, a strategic focus on generating reliable science and insights about effective care will finally occur; otherwise, we are sure to make major errors and endure major inefficiencies in serving the dying, all the while increasing their suffering and ours.

An Agenda for Change: Ideas to Include

What might work to make the last part of life as comfortable and meaningful as possible, at a cost that the community can sustain? Some elements might include the following.

- Articulate thresholds of severity of illness that indicate the onset of serious illness that is expected to last until death.
- From that time on, focus on care arrangements that stay with the patient and family across time and settings and that are comprehensive across all care needs.
- Insist on high standards of symptom prevention and relief, family support, and treatment and care planning.
- Pay sustainable salaries and decent benefits for paid workers, including home health aides and nursing assistants.
- Develop supports for family caregivers, such as health and disability insurance, adequate retirement security, respite care, and work to create a community that honors and respects the work of family caregivers.

- Develop an adequate supply of all of the critical components of good care, including hands-on services for personal care as well as hospital care, and good nursing homes as well as on-call nurses to handle crises in home care.
- Monitor the effectiveness and efficiency of innovative approaches, and deliberately replicate successful ones, aiming to evolve a highly reliable, sustainable care system within a decade.
- Do the research needed to enable reliable symptom relief.

In a way, this reform would dramatically expand hospice principles of continuity, patient and family focus, and care at home. It would also build on the social supports needed in home and institutional long-term care. It would limit the sense that patients must give up on treatment to get good care but would still make it unlikely to use burdensome treatments of limited value. The costs are probably not greatly different, though the priorities are.

WHY CAN'T WE DO THIS BY NEXT TUESDAY?

What gets in the way of doing this? First, of course, many powerful interests have a substantial investment in perpetuating the current system's dysfunctions. Those who lobbied for a broad prescription drug medication benefit under Medicare are not likely to have the same interest in lobbying for good working conditions for nursing home aides or for strategies that reduce the use of hospitals. Who could advocate for a more reasonable balance? The answer, tellingly, is that other than national hospice organizations, no strong industry interests are aligned with good care for the final phase of life. The professional trade associations that might seem to be likely candidates often give priority to their own particular interests, not to the general interests of dying patients and families.

The only group that comes to the fore as a potent force for thoughtful reform is comprised of family caregivers and policymakers. Almost all people have been, will be, or currently are family caregivers. They could take on a new identity as a political force and demand that industry and political leadership focus on their issues. That is a daunting claim—to take a diverse group that now has no particular self-identification, convince them that they have shared interests, and see them forge a political agenda and carry it through. Hope lies in the fact that the alternative is so distasteful—wasteful, unreliable services that also bankrupt the country and demoralize family members—and that all of us face this fate together, across the entire range of wealth and family structures.

In the meantime, you and your colleagues, people devoted to improving care at the final phase of life, are the only real advocates for patients and their loved ones. The dying themselves often cannot be a voice for change and improvement, and families caught up in caregiving or bereavement seldom have the energy or resources. But people who routinely work with dying patients, who see what eases their suffering and what worsens it, can offer the most compelling voice for change.

We are not suggesting that you become a lobbyist or change your day job, only that you use what you know to communicate with others in your organization and community—with your elected and appointed government officials, with program administrators and insurance officials—and tell them what needs to change and why and then suggest what might be done by the next election.

Tools and Resources

- Americans for Better Care of the Dying
  http://www.abcd-caring.org
- Lynn, J. (2004). *Sick to Death and Not Going to Take It Anymore! Reforming Health Care for the Last Years of Life.* Berkeley: University of California Press. Also available at http://www.medicaring.org

INDEX

advance care planning
overview, 43–45
aim statements, 45–47
barriers, 54–55
challenges, 44
and caregiver support, 100–101
change identification and testing, 50–55
communication strategies, 57–59
data displays, 50, 51
measurement strategies, 48–50
problem identification, 44–47
tools and resources, 56, 60
spreading the improvements, 55–60
team selection, 47–48
advanced dementia. *See* dementia care
advance directives, 3–4, 44
adverse-effect measures
generally, 30–31
advance care planning, 50
caregiver support, 106, 108
continuity of care, 123–124, 126
end-of-life care, 241
heart and lung failure, 143
hospice program quality, 228
intensive care units, 195–196
pain management, 64, 66–67
symptom management, 81–82, 84
aim statements
generally, 21–24, 28, 30–31, 34–35
advance care planning, 45–46
caregiver support, 97–99, 178–179

continuity of care, 119–121
dementia care, 174–180
end-of-life care, 236–239
heart and lung failure, 139–140
hospice program quality, 222–226
intensive care units, 192–193, 195–196
nursing home quality, 154–159
pain management, 62–63, 65–66
symptom management, 79–82
writing, how to, 23–24
See also measurement strategies

bereavement, 102, 107, 235, 243
tools and resources, 247
See also end-of-life care

cancer
pain statistics, 62
in trajectories model, 16–17, 253–254
cardiovascular disease. *See* heart and lung failure
caregiver support
overview, 95–97
aim statements, 97–100, 178–179
barriers, 100–102
change identification and testing, 99–100, 110, 112–115
data displays, 109–110
measurement strategies, 103–108
problem identification, 97–100

caregiver support (*continued*)
  tools and resources, 115
  spreading the improvements,
      112–115
  team selection and building, 102–
      103
  See also end-of-life care
Center to Advance Palliative Care
      (CAPC), 5, 6, 206, 210, 220
change identification and testing
  generally, 31–35
  advance care planning, 50–55
  caregiver support, 110, 112–115
  continuity of care, 127, 129–131
  dementia care, 185–186
  end-of-life care, 243–247
  heart and lung failure, 146–148
  hospice program quality, 228–231
  intensive care units, 198–202
  nursing home quality, 165–167
  pain management, 69–75
  symptom management, 85–89
  See also spreading the
      improvements
change maintenance, generally, 37–39
chronic conditions. *See* heart and
      lung failure
Closing the Quality Chasm, 4
cognitively-impaired patients,
      symptom management,
      88–89
comfort care. *See* symptom
      management
communicating the improvements.
      See data displays; spreading
      the improvements
consult services model, palliative
      care programs, 212–213
content experts, selecting, 25
continuity of care
  overview, 117–119
  aim statements, 119–121
  barriers, 121–122
  change identification and testing,
      127, 129–131

data displays, 127, 128
  defined, 118
  measurement strategies, 123–126
  palliative care programs and, 216
  problem identification, 119–121
  tools and resources, 135
  spreading the improvements,
      131–134
  strategies for, 133–134
  team selection, 122–123

data displays
  generally, 35–37
  advance care planning, 50, 51
  caregiver support, 109–110
  continuity of care, 127, 128
  dementia care, 186–188
  end-of-life care, 242–243
  heart and lung failure, 144–146
  hospice program quality, 228–229
  intensive care units, 196–198
  nursing home quality, 165
  pain management, 67–68
  symptom management, 84–85
dedicated inpatient model, palliative
      care programs, 212–213
dementia, in trajectories model, 16–
      18, 254
dementia care
  overview, 173–174
  aim statements, 174–180
  change identification and testing,
      185–186
  data displays, 186–188
  measurement strategies, 181–185
  problem identification, 174–180
  tools and resources, 189
  spreading the improvements,
      188–189
  team selection, 180–181
depression, prevention services
      project, 4
depression, symptom management, 93
diagnostic tests, pain control project,
      4–5

disease management, 138
   CHF/COPD, 147
displaying data. *See* data displays
durable powers of attorney for
   health care (DPOAHC), 44
dying, defining, 12–13
   "good death", 233–234
   See also end-of-life care; hospice
     entries

end-of-life care
   overview, 233–236
   aim statements, 236–239
   change identification and testing,
     243–247
   data displays, 242–243
   measurement strategies, 240–242
   policy, 255–257
   problem identification, 236–
     239
   tools and resources, 247
   team selection, 239–240

falls, prevention services project, 4
financing, palliative care programs,
   215
"frequent fliers," 120

healthcare system, improving. *See*
   public policies
heart and lung failure
   overview, 137–138
   aim statements, 139–140
   advance care planning for, 149–
     150
   barriers, 148–150
   change identification and testing,
     146–148
   data displays, 144–146
   improvement strategies, 147–148
   measurement strategies, 142–144
   medication kits for home, 151–
     152
   problem identification, 139–140
   tools and resources, 151–152

spreading the improvements,
   150–151
   team selection, 141–142
hospice
   limitations, 251, 254
   palliative care compared, 13–14
   and palliative care programs, 215–
     216
   staffing example, 5
hospice program quality
   overview, 221–222
   aim statements, 222–226
   change identification and testing,
     228–231
   data displays, 228–229
   measurement strategies, 227–228
   problem identification, 222–224
   tools and resources, 231–232
   team selection, 226–227

identifying potential changes. *See*
   change identification and
   testing
identifying problems. *See* problem
   identification
illness trajectories, models of, 14–18,
   252–255
improvement experts, selecting, 25
inpatient bed model, palliative care
   programs, 212–213
Institute of Medicine, six aims, 7
intensive care units
   overview, 191–192
   aim statements, 192–193, 195–196
   barriers, 202–203
   change identification and testing,
     198–202
   data displays, 196–198
   interdisciplinary care teams, 111–
     112
   measurement strategies, 195–196
   problem identification, 192–193
   spreading the improvements,
     204
   team selection, 194

interventions. *See* change
    identification and testing;
    spreading the improvements

leader selection, team, 25–26

maintaining changes, generally, 37–
    39
meal-delivery program, prevention
    services project, 4
measurement strategies
    generally, 28–31, 34–35
    advance care planning, 48–50
    caregiver support, 103–108
    continuity of care, 123–126
    dementia care, 181–185
    end-of-life care, 240–242
    heart and lung failure, 142–144
    hospice program quality, 227–228
    intensive care units, 195–196
    nursing home quality, 160–164
    pain management, 64–67
    palliative care programs, 217–219
    symptom management, 81–84
    See also aim statements
Medicare, hospice benefit, 13, 254
Medicare-developed tools and
    resources, 160
Meier, Diane, 210–211

nursing home quality
    overview, 153–154
    aim statements, 154–159
        for prevention, 156
        for wound healing, 156–157
    change identification and testing,
        165–169
    data displays, 165
    measurement strategies, 160–164
        for prevention, 161–162
        for healing, 162
        tools for lesions, 162
    problem identification, 154–159
    tools and resources, 170–171
        Medicare-developed, 160

spreading the improvements,
    169–170
    team selection, 159–160
NOPPAIN, 183

older patients, symptom
    management, 88–89
    palliative care, 209
    transisitons, 118
organization leaders, selecting, 25
organ systems failure, in trajectories
    model, 16–17, 254
outcome measures
    generally, 28–29, 31
    advance care planning, 49–50
    caregiver support, 105, 107–108
    continuity of care, 123–124, 126
    dementia care, 182–183
    end-of-life care, 241
    heart and lung failure, 142–143
    hospice program quality, 227–228
    intensive care units, 195–196
    pain management, 64–67
    palliative care programs, 217–219
    symptom management, 81–84
outpatient clinic model, palliative
    care programs, 212–213

PAIN AD, 183
pain management
    overview, 61–62
    aim statements, 62–63, 65–66
    barriers, 61, 71–72
    change identification and testing,
        69–75
    cognitively-impaired patients, 88–
        89
    data displays, 64, 67–68
    diagnostic tests project, 4–5
    improvement strategies, 61–62, 63
    measurement strategies, 64–67
    nonpharmacologic methods, 73
    older patients, 88–89
    opiod side effects, 74
    problem identification, 62–63

tools and resources for, 75–76
spreading the improvements, 72–
75
team selection, 63–64
palliative care
defined, 13–14, 206–207
and definitions of dying, 12–13
hospice compared, 13–14, 207
and trajectories model, 14–18
palliative care programs, building
overview, 205–211
assessment stage, 211–212
barriers to, 216–217
benefits of, 207, 210–211
financing, 215
growth planning, 219
hospice relationships, 215–216
measurement strategies, 217–219
tools and resources for, 220
staffing, 214
types of, 212–214
pressure sores. *See* nursing home
quality
pressure ulcers. *See* nursing home
quality
problem identification
generally, 22–23
advance care planning, 44–47
caregiver support, 97–99
continuity of care, 119–121
dementia care, 174–180
end-of-life care, 236–239
heart and lung failure, 139–140
hospice program quality, 222–224
intensive care units, 192–193
nursing home quality, 154–159
pain management, 62–63
symptom management, 79–81
process measures
generally, 29–30, 31
advance care planning, 49
caregiver support, 105, 106–107
continuity of care, 123–126
end-of-life care, 241–242
heart and lung failure, 142–143

hospice program quality, 228
intensive care units, 195–196
pain management, 64, 66–67
symptom management, 82–83
promises and improvement
priorities, 11–12
public policies
overview, 249–253
change possibilities, 255–257
tools and resources, 250, 257
trajectories model, 252–255
pulmonary disease. *See* heart and
lung failure; symptom
management
Pulse team. *See* heart and lung
failure
PUSH Tool, 162–164

quality improvement (QI) projects,
overview
assessing for, 8–12
benefits of, 6–7, 18–19
examples, 3–5
target areas, 6–7
and trajectories model, 15–18
quality improvement (QI) projects,
procedures
overview, 21–22, 41
aim statements, 23–24
change identification and testing,
31–35
data displays, 35–37
maintaining changes, 37–39
measurement strategies, 28–31
problem identification, 22–23
spreading the improvements, 39–
41
team selection, 24–27

rapid-cycle approach. *See* quality
improvement *entries*
Red Folder, 132
advance care planning, 56, 60
caregiver support, 115
continuity of care, 135

Red Folder (*continued*)
    dementia care, 189
    end-of-life care, 247
    hospice program quality, 222,
        231–232
    intensive care, 200
    nursing home quality, 162, 170–
        171
    pain management, 75–76
    palliative care programs, 206,
        220
    public policies, 250, 257
    symptom management, 94
run charts, 35–37
    See also data displays

spreading the improvements
    generally, 39–41
    advance care planning, 55–60
    caregiver support, 112–115
    continuity of care, 131–134
    dementia care, 188–189
    heart and lung failure, 150–151
    intensive care units, 204
    nursing home quality, 169–170
    pain management, 72–75
    symptom management, 90
    See also change identification and
        testing; data displays
staffing
    bereavement support for, 112–113
    career advancement, 112
    hospice project example, 5
    palliative care programs, 214
    See also team selection
storyboards, 35–37
    See also data displays
    surprise question, 13
"surprise question," defined, 13
symptom management
    overview, 77–79
    aim statements, 79–81
    barriers, 87–88
    best practices, 77–78
        for end of life, 78

    for older patients and
        cognitively impaired, 88–89
    change identification and testing,
        85–89
    data displays, 84–85
    maintaining the changes, 90
    measurement strategies, 81–84
    methods of, 90–93
    problem identification, 79–81
    resources for, 90–94
    spreading the improvements, 90
    team selection, 81–82

team selection
    generally, 24–27
    advance care planning, 47–48
    caregiver support, 102–103
    continuity of care, 122–123
    dementia care, 180–181
    end-of-life care, 239–240
    heart and lung failure, 141–142
    hospice program quality, 226–
        227
    intensive care units, 194
    nursing home quality, 159–160
    pain management, 63–64
    symptom management, 81–82
testing changes. *See* change
    identification and testing
time series graphs, generally, 35–37
    See also data displays
time-limited trials
    discuss with patients, 199–200
    intensive care unit and, 191
    invasive technology, 53, 56, 105
    medication and , 75
    sedation and, 143, 150
    ventilator and, 150
trajectories model, 14–18, 252–255
transfers. *See* continuity of care

ventilator withdrawal, 200–202
von Gunten, Charles, 212

Wong-Baker Scale, 70